Practical Research:
A Guide for Therapists

Skills for Practice Series

Series editors: Sally French and Jo Laing

Titles published

In preparation

Practical Research:
A Guide for Therapists

Sally French

BSc, MSc (Psych), MSc (soc), GradDip Phys, Dip.T.P.
Lecturer, School of Health, Welfare and Community
Education, Open University, UK

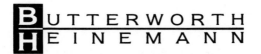

Butterworth-Heinemann Ltd
Linacre House, Jordan Hill, Oxford OX2 8DP

ℛ A member of the Reed Elsevier group

OXFORD   LONDON   BOSTON
MUNICH   NEW DELHI   SINGAPORE   SYDNEY
TOKYO   TORONTO   WELLINGTON

First published 1993

British Library Cataloguing in Publication Data
French, Sally
   Practical Research: A Guide for Therapists.
   – (Skills for Practice Series)
   I. Title II. Series
   001.40246158

ISBN 0 7506 0618 5

Library of Congress Cataloguing in Publication Data
French, Sally.
   Practical research: a guide for therapists/by Sally French.
   p.   cm. – (Skills for practice series)
   Includes bibliographical references and index.
   ISBN 0 7506 0618 5
   1. Medicine – Research – Methodology. 2. Physical therapy –
   Research – Methodology. I. Title. II. Series.
   [DNLM: 1. Research – methods.   2. Physical Therapy – methods.
   3. Writing.   WB 25 F876p 1993]
   R850.F684   1993
   615.8′2′072–dc20
                                                    93–14002
                                                    CIP

Printed and bound in Great Britain by Biddles Ltd, Guildford

Contents

vi   Contents

Preface

Over the past few years therapists and therapy students have become more involved in research, either as part of their degree studies, or as a way of improving their practice. The need to justify professional practice and demonstrate the efficiency of clinical interventions has always been important, but has become more urgent of late as health care practices and the use of resources have come under closer scrutiny. The theory and practice of the therapy professions encompass a wide range of diverse disciplines, ranging from physics and physiology to sociology and philosophy. It follows from this that if research within the therapy professions is to be comprehensive and meaningful, it needs to embrace a wide range of methods and approaches.

The aim of this book is to provide a broad and practical account of the many research methods and approaches which are available to therapists, ranging from those which are highly structured and quantitative, to those which are qualitative and open ended. It is emphasized throughout that no one method has a monopoly on 'the truth', but rather that each uncovers a particular type of knowledge. Ethical issues, the writing of research proposals and reports and the dissemination of research findings are also discussed.

Every effort has been made to ensure that the book is accessible to students and practitioners with no previous research knowledge or experience. It should also be useful to more practised researchers who are keen to extend their expertise in new directions. The book is extensively referenced to assist those readers who require further information.

I would like to thank all those who have helped, and who continue to help, me develop my research skills and knowledge. These include Nigel Goldie, Marianne Jaeger, Susan Lonsdale, Leon Gold, and all who have participated in my research. Thanks are also extended to Caroline Makepeace for her constant encouragement, faith and good humour, and to Jan Cox who taught me to use my computer. I am also grateful to *Therapy Weekly* for publishing a range of my articles in 1987 and 1988 which form the basis of some of the chapters in this book.

Most importantly of all, I would like to thank the many physiotherapy and nursing students I have taught, without whose challenges, insights and encouragement over the years I would never have developed the expertise or the confidence to write this book.

Sally French

Part One

Starting Research

1

Introduction to Research

Many people are almost as reluctant to undertake a piece of real research as they might be to do brain surgery. Yet doing research involves steps and skills which are no more complicated than many of the things that the average person can do easily, such as navigating from one side of the city to another, keeping a household budget, playing bridge or gardening. (Kane 1985:11)

What is research?

There is a great deal of mystique surrounding the process of doing research. Some people think it is an 'ivory tower' activity, divorced from everyday life and everything familiar, while others believe it is all about statistics, complicated computer packages and peering down microscopes. Kane (1985) reminds us, however, that we are all engaged in research throughout our lives. If, for example, we decide to go on an unfamiliar journey, we need to research what mode of transport to use, whether we are allowing sufficient time for our connections, what sort of ticket to buy, and whether we will reach our destination at a suitable time. Bailey defines research as 'any activity undertaken to increase our knowledge . . . It is the systematic investigation of a problem, issue or question' (1991:1). Thus, provided we do not carry out our travel investigations in a haphazard way, we can be said to be doing research. Most of us would agree, however, that in our everyday lives we do not observe or behave as systematically as those who are actively engaged in research.

Why do research?

Research is primarily undertaken because there is a need to further our knowledge. For some time therapists have been under intense pressure to demonstrate that their interventions are beneficial to patients and clients, as well as effective in terms of time and cost. Research has the potential to initiate more effective clinical practice and policy decisions, although it must be appreciated that it is enmeshed within social and political forces which are often outside therapists' control. This may mean that research findings are ignored or minimized because, for example, they oppose a fundamental belief of the profession, would cause great upheaval to implement, or would challenge the views or work of an influential member.

A further important reason why therapists should do research is to enable them to evaluate the research of others. Although it is possible to learn about research procedures from books, there is no quicker or more effective way to understand them than to become actively involved. This learning process is often initiated when therapists undertake research as part of a degree programme.

It is probably true to say that interest and curiosity lie at the heart of most research endeavours; if they are absent it will be very difficult for the researcher to tolerate the set-backs and drudgery that the research process inevitably entails. It is also important that researchers can relate to the topic they have chosen to study. Whatever the motive for undertaking research, it is essential to ensure that the interests of the research participants are kept centrally in mind. Disabled people, for example, have complained that much of the research carried out about them has failed to reflect their perspectives and concerns. It can also be argued that doing research *purely* for interest or to satisfy curiosity is unethical.

Research methods

Different subject disciplines, or schools of thought within disciplines, focus on particular research methods. This is, to some extent, grounded in their history, but mainly reflects the type of knowledge which they seek. Thus those involved in the 'hard' sciences (physiology, physics, chemistry, etc.), where causal relationships between specific factors are sought, use experimental methods of research, whereas anthropologists, who immerse themselves in the communities they study in order to gain the in-depth knowledge they require, tend to use unstructured observation as their major research method. No research method can be said to monopolise 'the truth'.

Research methods are often deeply embedded within particular theories, which in turn are associated with different schools of philosophy or ways of looking at the world (Parry 1991). If, for example, a team of therapists studying the causes of illness in poor people are of the opinion that their health status results from malfunctional behaviour, their research is likely to focus on that behaviour, and the methods they use will, in turn, reflect the theory within which they are working. If, on the other hand, they believe that the health status of poor people results from factors outside their control, such as the way in which society is ordered in terms of employment, housing and the distribution of wealth, then their research will focus on these wider social structures, which again will influence their choice of research method.

Research methods can also go in and out of fashion as ideas change and as various merits or shortcomings are either highlighted or ignored. Such changes are often influenced by wider social and political factors. The case study, for example, was the major research method used in psychology until the 1950s when it fell into disrepute and was superseded by experimental research as psychology attempted to emulate the 'hard' sciences. Since then experimental research within psychology has been strongly criticised for its artificiality, and the case study has experienced something of a revival. Similarly, in the 1960s there was a reaction against survey research in sociology, and a move towards participant observation which, it was felt, provided deeper and more meaningful knowledge of human behaviour.

There are many ways of categorizing research. One of the most frequent categorizations is that of 'quantitative' and 'qualitative' research, although in reality research methods and approaches can be placed on a continuum from quantitative to qualitative. Quantitative research is associated with experimentation, statistics and 'objectivity', whereas qualitative research is 'fundamentally concerned with meaning, understanding and subjective reality' (Stone 1991:449). In quantitative research the theory is already formulated and the researcher seeks to verify it, whereas in qualitative research theory may emerge as the research progresses, that is the study structures the research rather than the other way round, giving rise to the notion of 'grounded theory' (Glaser and Srauss 1967). Siddell states:

> Qualitative methods arise from a different philosophical tradition, one which looks for meaning behind social action. This involves more than observing the social world, it requires interaction with the social world. As researcher you must be part of the process, you need to understand the symbolic nature of social action in the search for meaning. (1993)

The therapy professions have been closely bound with the medical profession and this has shaped the methods used in therapy research in favour of quantification. Only in recent times has qualitative research been respected and advocated as a suitable way of investigating the therapy professions (Stone 1991).

Although quantitative research is said to be 'objective', it is important not to be fooled by pages of impressive looking tables and diagrams as they are no guarantee of unbiased or impartial research. More fundamentally, it can be argued that objectivity is impossible because however impartial research may seem, it is inevitably shaped by the perceptions and perspectives of the researchers undertaking it, which in turn are shaped by the culture, time and place of which they are a part. (Irvine *et al.* 1979, French 1988a). As Laing points out:

> scientists sometimes forget that it is by the aid of non-objective mental operations that we switch to being objective – non-objective changes bring into view the objective world. (1983:17)

Even the most objective looking research from the past can appear quaint when viewed from the perspective of our particular culture and place in history, for events can only be fully understood when they are situated within their social and historical context. Who the researchers are, within any given society, also influences the interpretation of research data. In the 1980s sociology saw the growth of feminist research which has demonstrated that many investigations have been disproportionately shaped by the perceptions and perspectives of men. Feminist researchers have succeeded in offering alternative interpretations of data and have highlighted the extent to which even the most 'hard-nosed' research is shaped by the perceptions and experiences of the researchers (McNeill 1990, Morris 1992, Williams 1993).

There has been a great deal of conflict and argument over which research methods should be used in any given discipline, but fortunately a stage has been reached where it is appreciated that no one method is 'better' or 'worse' than another. As Parry puts it:

> the differences do not necessarily mean that one is superior to the other or that they are in competition with each other. We need only understand that different styles of research reveal different kinds of useful information. (1991:437)

A wide variety of methods are needed to help us understand the complexities of human behaviour. It may be useful, for example, to carry out some quantitative research to discover how many patients fail to attend for their entire course of treatment, or how many patients are successfully rehabiliated following spinal cord injury, but this research will be of limited value unless we also understand *why* patients fail to complete their treatment programmes or whether patients with spinal injuries *agree* that their rehabilitation has been a success. These are questions which can best be answered by qualitative research.

Quantitative and qualitative research can be mutually enhancing. Qualitative research may allow the researcher to give meaning to quantitative data, and quantitative data may help to put qualitative research into a wider context. If both point to the same conclusions the validity of the research will be enhanced, and if, on the other hand, there are discrepancies this may lead to further questions and further development of theory. As Siddell (1993) states, 'Research frequently throws up more questions than it answers and in so doing manages to perpetuate the process'.

Combining quantitative and qualitative methods may not, however, always be straightforward for, as noted above, the methods are often linked to specific ways of viewing the world which may be diametrically opposed. As Anzul points out, 'Most of us have come to qualitative research with attitudes towards "objectivity" and "subjectivity" as part of our cultural baggage' (1991:220). Bryman (1988) notes that if quantitative and qualitative methods are combined they are rarely given equal weight. (For further details of the quantitative/qualitative debate, readers are referred to Bryman 1988.)

Choosing a research method

There are many ways of investigating a topic, and the method or methods used should reflect the research questions posed. Sometimes research methods, be they questionnaires, interviews or experiments, assume such importance in the minds of researchers that they attempt to fit their questions into the methods rather than choosing appropriate methods to fit their questions. As Stone remarks, 'The methods used are important only in terms of how well they enable the goal of the research to be reached and are not ends in themselves' (1991:449). If, for example, a team of therapists wanted to investigate the ways in which working-class Victorians coped with illness, they would probably carry out a detailed historical literature review. If, on the other hand, they wanted to discover the attitudes of adolescents to disabled people, they would probably choose to undertake an interview or questionnaire study. The group under consideration may also dictate the methods used, for example a postal questionnaire is not suitable for use with young children.

There is frequently more than one appropriate method which can be chosen. The choice will often depend on the precise research question posed. For example if the researcher requires detailed, in-depth information from participants, then the interview is likely to be a more successful method than the questionnaire. There are also many practical considerations which need to be taken into account when choosing a method, such as the amount of time and money available to carry out the research, ethical considerations, and whether it is possible to gain direct access to the people under investigation. It is sometimes impossible for researchers to use the methods they consider most suitable.

It is unfortunate that particular methods are sometimes chosen simply because they are the only ones with which the researcher is familiar. As Bryman states:

> Because researchers are often trained in the ways of particular styles of research, their ability and inclination to flirt with other approaches is often limited . . . Thus a researcher who is inclined towards survey methods is likely to routinely formulate his or her research problem in such a way that it will be amenable to a survey approach; he or she does not decide the problem and then select the appropriate method. (1988:154)

There is no ideal or perfect method, and if time and resources allow it is wise with most studies of human behaviour to use more than one method. For too long therapists have felt obliged to use only quantitative, so-called 'objective' methods, but recently a change of attitude has become apparent. Stone believes that:

> One thing that has to be accepted is that there is no single perfect way to understand human health and behaviour. If it were that simple many problems would have been solved by now. It is thus important that any growing profession should be liberated to be imaginative in its outlook to research and flexible in the methods it is prepared to try. (1991:451)

It is now becoming widespread practice to use several methods of research when complex issues are investigated. (For further information of the multi-method approach, readers are referred to Chapter 14.)

Reliability and validity

Whatever research method is adopted, it is important to consider whether or not the research instruments and procedures used are reliable and valid. The aim of this section is to explain these important concepts in general terms. Issues of reliability and validity, pertaining to specific research instruments and procedures, will be discussed throughout this book.

Reliability

> Reliability is the extent to which a test or procedure produces similar results under constant conditions on all occasions. (Bell 1987:50)

An instrument or procedure is unreliable under the following conditions:

1. If the researcher arrives at different measurements when measuring the same entity on different days.
2. If different researchers fail to agree when measuring the same entity.
3. If research participants give disparate answers on different occasions when working through the same test.

If the measurements and procedure used in research are unreliable, then the validity of the research is seriously threatened. Just as we are unlikely to have much faith in a clock which loses on some days and gains on others, or on a bus that is sometimes early and at other times late, we cannot rely on unreliable research instruments or procedures.

There are three main ways of testing the reliability of a measurement.

1. Test–retest

Research participants who have completed a test are given the same test after a lapse of time. If their results are very similar on both occasions the test is reliable. The interval of time between giving the tests should be far enough apart to prevent participants remembering their responses to the first test, but not so far apart that their scores might be affected by extraneous factors.

2. Equivalent forms (alternate forms, parallel forms)

Two equivalent, but different, versions of the same test are given to research participants on the same occasion, and the scores are correlated. The greater the positive correlation between the two sets of scores (i.e. their similarity), the more reliable the test.

3. Split halves (inter-consistency reliability)

If the items on a test are measuring the same entity, for example intelligence or compliance, it can be split into two equal halves and correlated when completed. The greater the positive correlation, the more reliable the test. The odd numbered items are usually correlated with the even numbered items; it is not a good idea to correlate the first half of the test with the second half, as erroneous effects, such as lack of concentration or tiredness on the part of participants during the second half of the test, may be introduced.

These methods are not without their problems. Choosing the right time interval for the test–retest method is difficult, and devising two versions of the same test is very complicated, especially as it is known that even small changes of wording can bring about altered responses. In addition, testing research participants on two separate occasions is often impracticable.

Several observations of the same research participant will improve reliability, as may testing participants at the same time of the day and by the same researcher. Meticulous recording and checking by researchers also improves reliability; it is well known that records, including medical records, can be notoriously unreliable. (Formal checking of reliability is not usually necessary in undergraduate research.)

Validity

> The validity of an instrument is the extent to which it measures what it is supposed to measure. (Berger and Patchner 1988a:68).

Determining validity is far more complicated than determining reliability, because whereas reliability is basically concerned with technicalities, validity is concerned with the nature of reality.

It is possible for a test to be highly reliable but, none the less, invalid. If, for example, a standard intelligence quotient (IQ) test is given to children with severe visual or hearing impairments, they may produce low scores in a highly reliable way, but this is unlikely to have anything to do with their level of intelligence. Similarly, reliable measures of joint range and muscle strength may have little to do with the ability of disabled people to live independently. Berger and Patchner (1988a) point out that although it is impossible to have a valid measure which is not reliable, it is possible to have a reliable measure which is not valid. You must be satisfied that your test is valid before concerning yourself with issues of reliability. As Plummer puts it, 'There is no point in being very precise about nothing' (1983:102).

Internal validity

According to Judd et al., internal validity concerns 'the extent to which conclusions can be drawn about the causal effects of one variable on another' (1991:28). In other words, internal validity is high if we can be sure that our intervention, rather than extraneous factors, brought about the effect. Simple correlations, for example the recovery of patients after receiving a certain type of therapy, thus have little internal validity.

External validity

External validity is concerned with the extent to which research findings can be generalized beyond the sample of research participants tested.

Judd *et al.* (1991) make the point that paying very close attention to maximizing internal validity can reduce external validity. Ensuring high internal validity can render conditions so contrived and artificial that they no longer relate to the real world. This is a criticism levelled against some laboratory research.

Some threats to validity

History

Concurrent events in the lives of research participants may be responsible for the changes observed. A patient may, for example, suddenly start to walk, not because of the treatment he or she has received, but because of the offer of a new ground floor flat.

Maturation

Developmental changes, taking place over a period of time, may have brought about the observed change, rather than the effects of the research procedures. For example, a child's speech may improve, not because of the speech and language therapy he or she has received, but simply because the child has matured.

Testing

Research participants may be affected by the actual testing procedures used. For example, they may get accustomed to particular tests, which helps them to perform at a higher standard; this is a criticism levelled against IQ tests. The placebo effect may also operate, influencing participants behaviour.

Unreliable instruments

Unreliable test instruments, for example questionnaires, thermometers or interview schedules, always threaten the validity of research.

Selection of participants

If a particular type of research participant is chosen, this may threaten internal validity by making it impossible for the researcher to infer causal relationships. If, for example, most of the children in a particular class come from crowded and poverty stricken families, their poor performance in examinations may have nothing to do with their school or with their intelligence. This problem can be reduced, if practicable and ethical, by randomly assigning research participants to different groups.

Knowledge and behaviour of participants

If the research is covert, for example if the researcher is secretly observing the participants, and they get to know of this, their knowledge may threaten the validity of the research. If, on the other hand, participants are taking part in the research against their wishes, they may deliberately give the wrong responses. If they are very anxious their performance may suffer, and if assurances of confidentiality are not provided they may omit vital information. All of these behavioural responses will threaten the validity of the research.

Participant mortality

The loss of research participants, as the research progresses, can lead to an unrepresentative sample, threatening the validity of the research. This can occur, for example, if only those participants with a personal interest in the topic under investigation, or only those with sufficient time, remain.

Interaction between the researcher and the research participants

Researchers and research participants inevitably influence each other. For example, the mood of the participant may affect the researcher, and the dress, race and gender of the researcher may affect the participant. All of these factors threaten to reduce the validity of the research (Rosenthal 1976, Silverman 1977).

Unrepresentative samples

If the sample is unrepresentative, researchers cannot generalize their findings to a wider population, reducing external validity.

Statistical regression

If people with very atypical pre-test scores are selected to receive a particular intervention, it is likely that their scores, being extreme, will be subject to more error than the scores of those who were not selected. Thus improvement with or without the intervention is more likely to occur in the referred group.

These and other threats to validity will be discussed throughout this book.

Types of validity

Face validity

Face validity refers to whether a test looks as if it is measuring what it professes to measure. Face validity is very subjective, and may not be sufficient, but researchers should always think long and hard about the measurements they use and seek expert help and comment. Involving research participants in the design of measurements and the analysis of data, may also improve validity.

Content validity

Content validity refers to whether or not the test covers a representative sample of items. When devising a questionnaire to measure job satisfaction, for example, it should express all aspects of that multi-faceted concept. As Rubin and Babbie put it, content validity 'refers to the degree to which a measure covers the range of meanings included within a concept' (1989:147).

Discriminate validity

A test can be said to have discriminate validity if it fails to correlate highly with tests which assess unrelated constructs.

Empirical validity (criterion validity)

Empirical validity concerns whether the test correlates with others claiming to measure the same entity. A new test of motor skills, for example, would have greater empirical validity if it correlated positively with other tests of motor skills.

Predictive validity

Predictive validity is a variant of empirical validity; it refers to the correlation between a measurement and subsequent behaviour relating to that measurement. If, for example, therapy students who perform well in practical examinations go on to practice the same techniques proficiently in the clinical situation, then the examinations can be said to have predictive validity.

Construct validity

Construct validity refers to the extent to which a test is measuring the underlying theoretical constructs. Judd *et al.* state:

A variable that has a great deal of construct validity is one that mostly measures the construct of interest, with minimal contribution of constructs of disinterest or random error. (1991:30)

Thus a multiple choice anatomy test with a high degree of construct validity will be one which tests students' knowledge of anatomy, rather than their memory (construct of disinterest) or their ability to guess the correct answers (random error).

Construct validity can be tested by measuring concepts in several different ways and then comparing the results. Thus if certain students tend to do well on tests of anatomy, regardless of the format of the tests, while other students tend to do poorly on all the tests, then the tests are high in construct validity. Brewer and Hunter state:

Measures that correlate highly only with methodologically similar measures may be reliable but their validity is doubtful because of the strong possibility of methodological bias. (1989:134)

Therapists should make every effort to improve the validity of the tests and instruments they use in research. Formally testing validity is, however, a daunting and time-consuming process which can become a major project in itself; it is rarely required of undergraduate researchers. There are many ways of improving the validity of tests and measurements, however, and these will be discussed throughout this book in relation to particular methods. For more detailed information on measuring validity, readers are referred to Kerlinger (1973), Anastasi (1976) and Thorndike and Hogan (1977). For more detailed information on reliability and validity in qualitative research, readers are referred to Kirk and Miller (1986).

Stages in the research process

When undertaking a research project, various stages must be worked through. These stages depend, to some extent, on the research methods used but they usually comply with the following sequence.

Stage 1. Identifying a problem to be investigated

This will involve thinking, talking and reading around the subject. It often arises through general experience.

Stage 2. Reviewing the literature

When the problem to be investigated is identified, it is necessary to review the existing literature pertaining to that particular problem. It is important that the reading is focused.

Stage 3. Defining the research question or hypothesis

The research question or hypothesis must be defined very precisely. If, for example, a therapist is interested in studying 'disruptive behaviour' following brain injury, there will be little chance of recording or measuring it unless the researcher has decided exactly what disruptive behaviour means (*see* Chapter 2).

Stage 4. Planning the research

At this stage the researcher should contact key people who may be of help in the investigation, for example a statistician or those whose permission must be sought to carry out the research or to gain access to the research participants. Research tools must also be devised, for example questionnaires or interview schedules, and the research procedures, for example how to contact research participants, how many participants to include in the research and how much time to allow for each stage of the research process, must be carefully planned. A research proposal may also need to be written for inspection by an ethics committee or to apply for funding (*see* Chapter 4).

Stage 5. Gathering the information

It is usually advisable to carry out a small pilot study before the 'real' study commences so that any problems that remain can be identified and eliminated or reduced. There may, for example, be an ambiguous question in the questionnaire, or the therapist may have underestimated the amount of time it will take to carry out a series of experiments.

Stage 6. Analysing the data

This is a major and exciting aspect of the research process which will vary according to the research methods used. It may, for example, involve a statistical analysis or a more open-ended evaluation.

Stage 7. Writing up the data

A major part of any research project is to write it up in such a way that it can be easily understood, digested and, if possible, replicated by other researchers.

State 8. Disseminating the data

This final stage of the research process is very often neglected, but research will have little value unless it is disseminated to others who may learn from it and act upon it.

Conclusion

The remaining chapters of this book will seek to explain the various stages of the research process. A wide variety of research methods and approaches which therapists may use to answer the questions which fascinate them, and which may help to enhance their practice, will be critically analysed.

Chapter

2

Developing Research Ideas

Arriving at a suitable idea or problem to be researched is often the most difficult stage of the entire research process. On occasions therapists may be obliged to undertake specific pieces of research, in which case decisions regarding the topic may not be their own, but more often than not they are expected to choose a topic themselves, perhaps as part of a course or as a way of enhancing their clinical practice.

Research ideas usually arise from a desire to know more about a topic. Such ideas can be activated by almost any situation: talking to colleagues, observing patients and clients, reading, listening, or watching the television. Therapists are constantly asking themselves questions as they go about their daily work: 'Why did Mr Clark's speech improve so much faster than Mr Smith's?'; 'Will those exercises I gave Mrs Jones really help?'; 'Why is it that Mr Singh is so much more enthusiastic about his rehabilitation than Mr Wood?' In discussing questions such as these with colleagues, or by searching the literature for further information, it often becomes apparent that gaps in the knowledge exist which could be bridged by further research. Asking 'Who?', 'Why?', 'What?', 'When?', 'Where?' and 'How?' of any topic can be a good way of generating research ideas.

It is vitally important that therapists choose research topics which they find both interesting and important. Personal commitment is essential to see researchers through the many problems that inevitably arise as the research project progresses, as well as the tedium of some of the work, like feeding lists of numbers into a computer or addressing hundreds of envelopes. Doing research may seem glamorous to those who have never been involved, but in reality it often consists of long periods of routine work interspersed with spells of great excitement.

Formulating a researchable question

There are several stages which researchers go through when formulating a researchable question.

1. Identifying a general problem area

Ideas usually arise in a very general, diffuse and ill-defined state where it is possible to think of many potential research topics which could ensue. The therapist may decide, for example, to study 'shoulder pain', 'patient compliance' or 'job satisfaction'. Except in the most qualitative of research methods, such wide and vague research areas would not be satisfactory. To take shoulder pain as an example, therapists would need to define precisely what they mean by 'pain' and how it can be measured. Does the pain relate to a specific disease or injury? Will patients within a particular age range be studied? From what theoretical perspective – physiological, psychological, sociological – will pain be examined? Some people find it useful at this early stage to elucidate their thinking by engaging in a 'brainstorming' session in which all their thoughts and ideas on the topic are written down. It may then be possible to organize the ideas into major themes which will begin to provide shape, clarity and greater focus to the topic.

2. Relating the problem to existing theory

Having identified a general problem area, the next step is to carry out a detailed literature review. This will enable researchers to obtain a sound understanding of any information which exists on the topic and to decide which areas need further investigation. It will also indicate the range of methods that have been used and how the results from previous studies have been interpreted. According to Berger and Patchner:

> A study should never be done in a vacuum, but should take place within the body of knowledge that currently exists. (1988b:51)

(For further information on undertaking a literature review, the reader is referred to Chapter 5.)

3. Narrowing the focus of the research problem

In narrowing the focus of the research problem, it is important that researchers decide and make clear the precise meanings of the concepts they intend to investigate. 'Health' and 'illness', for example, can mean many things to many people; such concepts must be unambiguous and clearly expressed. Partridge and Barnitt state that 'If a word or expression cannot be defined it cannot be researched' (1986:13), and Kane believes that 'Failure to define major research words is probably the most important mistake made by researchers' (1985:17). Kane goes on to warn that if researchers use a broad, general word they are responsible for studying all of its aspects! The concepts which words symbolize are usually so complex that their everyday meanings are insufficient when undertaking research.

It can be very helpful at this stage to list the aims and objectives of the study and to state, very briefly, what it is about. Although ideas are bound to change as the research progresses, it is an excellent way for researchers to clarify their thoughts and to specify a problem which is manageable and amenable to research.

4. Devising operational definitions

Operational definitions refer to the procedures and operations researchers must go through to measure the concepts they wish to investigate. In order to measure pain, for example, the concept may be broken down into 'intensity', 'type' and 'duration', and suitable scales, tick lists and questions devised. Similarly, 'intelligence' may be defined in terms of various verbal, spatiial and mathematical abilities which are measured by tets of IQ.

The more abstract the concept, the more difficult it is to arrive at a satisfactory operational definition. 'Range of movement' and 'muscle strength', for example, are far easier to operationalize than 'anxiety' and 'depression'. Operational definitions must be related to theoretical concepts, but they are not the same, as they are far more specific. With abstract concepts it is usually necessary to devise multi-faceted measures. One indicator of 'patient compliance', for example, might be regular attendance for therapy, but that is unlikely, in itself, to tell us very much; patients may, for example, be forced to attend by their parents or spouses, but may none the less totally reject the advice they are given by the therapist.

The operational definitions arrived at may well have far reaching consequences. If, for example, a therapist attempts to measure the success of a treatment programme, the outcome of the study will depend to a large extent on how 'success' is defined. Operational definitions can be very significant politically; the ways in which poverty or disability are defined and operationalized, for example, dictate how many people are disabled and how much poverty exists. This, in turn, is likely to have consequences regarding the extent to which people are entitled to various state benefits. This emphasizes very clearly how research, even at its most 'objective', is shaped by the ideas and perceptions of researchers and powerful people within society.

5. Stating hypotheses or research questions

Researchers need to state clearly and concisely their overall research questions or hypotheses. A hypothesis is a theory which is put forward for testing in order that it can be accepted or rejected. Hypothesis testing is particularly associated with experimental research and will be discussed in more detail in Chapter 11. Therapists' hypotheses may include:

1. Patients from professional backgrounds are more compliant.
2. Shoulder pain is experienced as less acute by people over 65.

Research questions, on the other hand, may include:

1. Does social class influence compliance?
2. Is age a factor in the experience of shoulder pain?

From the formulation of a very broad and ill-defined research problem, the researcher has arrived at specific research questions or hypotheses and has the tools of measurement available to move the research to the next phase.

Conclusion

For convenience and clarity the process of developing research ideas has been considered in sequential steps, but in reality this is rarely how it happens. When, for example, the research problem becomes focused, it may be necessary to return to the literature; similarly, when operational definitions have been formulated, the focus of the research may narrow or broaden. During the entire research process new insights and ideas are likely to develop which may have implications for all the work that has been done. As was noted in Chapter 1, when using some qualitative methods it is both legitimate and desirable to allow the research questions and the theory to emerge as the research progresses.

Arriving at researchable problems and questions is difficult and time consuming and there can be an understandable tendency to rush into later stages of the research too soon. Attending to the development of ideas is, however, time well spent, as it clarifies thinking and helps to avoid difficulties arising later on; in addition it makes the nature of the research clear to others and may enable them to replicate the study.

3

Ethical Issues

Homan (1991) describes ethics as 'the science of morality', with those engaging in it determining values for the regulation of behaviour. Ethical questions and dilemmas permeate the entire research process, from the formulation of aims to the publication and dissemination of findings, and involve everyone involved in research, however peripheral their involvement may be. As Sim states:

> Ethics in research is not a discrete entity but a 'conceptual framework' which underpins and permeates virtually every feature of the research process. (Sim 1989:237)

Whether or not we do research is, in itself, an ethical issue, for we cannot really judge the effectiveness of our treatment procedures without it. As Judd *et al.* state, 'A decision not to act when the action is warranted, is as morally reprehensible as a decision to act when action is not warranted' (1991:481). Poorly designed research can also be regarded as unethical as it may give rise to false data which, in turn, could be harmful to individuals, as well as hindering knowledge.

The aim of this chapter is to highlight the major ethical questions and dilemmas with which researchers are faced. Ethical issues pertaining to particular research methods and approaches will be discussed throughout this book.

Research ethics and research participants

Respect

The welfare of research participants should always be at the front of the researcher's mind. It is easy, especially for experienced researchers investigating groups, to view them as objects rather than people with feelings and rights. As Judd *et al*. explain:

> A given research participant is one among many persons whose thoughts and actions are studied in a single project. One consequence is an insidious tendency to treat the participants as research objects and to forget their human sensitivities. (1991:512)

This can occur in small but important ways, such as arriving late for interviews, or failing to send a promised summary of the findings.

An area of concern with regard to the respect of research participants, is research designed to alter their behaviour. It can be argued that researchers have no right to attempt this, even if the behaviour change is judged to be desirable. On the other hand, behaviour modification is claimed to be legitimate if it is undertaken for the person's own welfare. Some researchers, in defence of behaviour modification, also stress that our behaviour is controlled within society by forces far stronger than those within research.

Informed consent

Partridge and Barnitt (1986) believe that research participants should give their informed consent, both verbally and in writing, before research proceeds. It is only possible to give informed consent if a full explanation of the research is provided. This should include:

1. The aims of the research.
2. The purpose of the research.
3. The identity of the researchers.

4. The nature of the institution where the research will be undertaken.
5. How the individual was selected.
6. Precisely what participation in the research entails.
7. To what use the research will be put.

Participants must also be assured that they have the right to ask questions and to opt out of the research at any time.

If participants are unable to give their informed consent, it may be obtained from a relative or guardian. The rights of vulnerable people, particularly those in institutions, must, however, be rigorously safeguarded. Sim states that 'the therapist should ensure that the interpersonal forces that operate in the therapeutic relationship are not used as a lever to secure participation in experimental procedures' (1986:586). If the research puts the participants at no physical or psychological risk, for example if they are asked to fill in an impersonal questionnaire, informed consent may not be necessary and is not usually obtained (Berger and Patchner 1988a).

Unfortunately, informed consent is not as straightforward as it may at first seem. With some research projects, validity may depend on the participants' ignorance of all, or at least some, aspects of procedures or intentions. As Judd et al. state, 'although a questionable practice may sometimes be eliminated, at other times to do so is tantamount to abandoning the proposed research' (1991:479). To tell participants they are receiving placebos, for example, is likely to invalidate the research.

Even the most respectable looking studies frequently contain some deception or other questionable practice. Educational research, for example, is frequently carried out without the knowledge or awareness of the students who are taking part, and the participation of students as research participants is sometimes a requirement of their courses. A neutral attitude to behaviour or ideas, which would normally cause anger or disapproval, can also be regarded as deceptive. Jenkins (1987) goes as far as to say that relationship building with interviewees is a 'cynical ploy' to improve the quality of the research data. In addition it is often impossible for researchers to give full information of their research; research procedures, particularly if the research is qualitative, tend to emerge as the research progresses, and the utilization of the research findings may be outside the researcher's control. Research methods and procedures do not, therefore, fall neatly into 'overt' or 'covert' categories, but are on a continuum where various aspects of the research vary from complete openness to complete secrecy.

As well as being an ethical issue, gaining informed consent also reduces legal liability and in that way protects the researcher. It can also be used as a means of obtaining access to research participants (Peace 1993).

One way round the problem of deception is to ask participants for their permission to be deceived. This is, however, likely to reduce the validity of the research, and may lead to a climate of suspicion and mistrust. Alternatively, an explanation of why the researcher found it necessary to deceive participants can be provided when their involvement in the research is over. Even though it is less scientifically rigorous, it is usually advisable to ask for volunteers rather than coerce people to take part in research.

Researching publicly accountable behaviour, is an area where researchers may feel it justifiable to deny research participants informed consent. Galliher (1973) believes that private roles should be safeguarded against covert research, but not public roles, where people should be accountable for their actions, and where they may be hiding information to suit their own vested interests. Many studies of discrimination against marginalized groups have used covert techniques as perhaps the only way of uncovering such behaviour.

Anonymity and confidentiality

Rubin and Babbie (1989) draw the distinction between anonymity and confidentiality in research. They state:

> A respondent may be considered anonymous when the researcher cannot identify a given response with a given respondent ... in a confidential survey the researcher is able to identify a given person's response but essentially promises not to do so publicly. (1989:53)

Participants often assume anonymity and confidentiality, and researchers should be careful not to exploit this.

Ensuring that anonymity and confidentiality is protected throughout the research process, and beyond, is far from easy. Changing the name and the gender of a person in a written report, for example, may not be enough and, in any event, opens up a new ethical issue, that of deception of the readership. Anonymity and confidentiality also extend beyond the written word to include photographs, video and audio recordings, and raw data. Coded information should always be kept well away from research data and destroyed when it is no longer needed.

Anonymity and confidentiality can be breached in many ways. Researchers may come under intense pressure, for example from parents, institutions or the courts, to release information. Information may be passed from one professional to another without the participant's knowledge or permission, or anonymity and confidentiality may be lost at the stage of publication and dissemination, where the researcher may lose influence and control. Researchers may occasionally hear alarming information from participants, for example that they are planning to commit suicide, and may feel under an obligation to breach their confidence and intervene. Anonymity and confidentiality may not always be in the best interests of research participants, however. They may, for example, be eager for publicity, especially if they believe it might bring about an improvement in their situation or give them personal recognition.

Homan (1991) points out that one of the major reasons for ensuring research participants of anonymity and confidentiality is to secure their co-operation. It also offers researchers some legal protection.

Privacy

Privacy may be invaded by many research methods. These include observation, questionnaire and interview questions, audio and video tapes, disguised tests, and obtaining information from a third party. Invasion of privacy violates a basic human right, but can also harm participants in more direct ways, for example by uncovering criminal behaviour.

The greater the sensitivity of the information the greater the need to protect the participant's privacy. Many researchers believe, however, that the invasion of privacy involved in most research projects is trivial when compared with the invasion of privacy experienced in our everyday lives.

Researchers must weigh up the benefits of carrying out the research against the costs to the research participants. As Kimmel states:

> a psychologist who refuses to do a study because it involves an invasion of subjects' privacy, but that, if conducted, might reduce violence or prejudice, has not solved an ethical problem, but has merely traded one problem for another. (1988:35)

The costs and benefits of *not* doing research must always be addressed.

Safety

It is important that researchers ensure that participants come to no harm during the research, either physically or psychologically; the prevention of harm is one of the reasons why medical ethical guidelines are so stringent. Behavioural or social research is unlikely to be as hazardous but, nevertheless, research participants may be caused unpleasant emotions, such as stress, guilt or a lowering of self-esteem, by the research procedures. For example, a researcher investigating honesty or altruism may provide research participants with opportunities to lie, cheat or 'pass by on the other side'. Participants must then go away with this new and unpleasant knowledge of themselves.

Some researchers believe that participants are responsible for their own behaviour, and that researchers may, in fact, be doing them a service by highlighting inadequacies. This is a weak argument, however, as exposing and changing behaviour is a sensitive process which often requires counselling.

Research participants may be harmed by adverse labelling, for example designating them 'non-compliant' or 'slow to improve' for the purposes of research. They may also be harmed by the indirect effects of research interventions. For example, a research procedure which succeeds in reducing the amount a person smokes may also increase that person's level of anxiety. Similarly, research aimed at detecting high blood pressure may lead those so discovered to change their behaviour in harmful ways. Some research may raise the consciousness of research participants to their own situation, for example to discrimination which may be limiting their lives. They may be very grateful for this, but, on the other hand, the newly found knowledge may create frustration, anger and dissatisfaction.

Research participants may also be harmed when research projects end; elderly people in an institution may, for example, have thoroughly enjoyed sharing their memories, week after week, with an oral historian, or a group of people with learning difficulties may have enjoyed the contact of a researcher attempting to change their behaviour. Once researchers withdraw, research participants may even regress.

These examples demonstrate the complexity of behaving ethically when undertaking research. As Kimmel states:

> The likelihood that multiple ethical questions will emerge within a given situation demonstrates how important it is for an investigator to maintain caution in attempting to isolate *the* ethical question with a single research problem. One also must be sensitive to the possible consequences of any action since a response to one aspect of any ethical dilemma may, at the same time, exacerbate or give rise to other unanticipated troublesome issues. (1988:31)

If research participants have been subject to deception, or any degree of stress, debriefing can avoid negative effects and restore trust. When debriefing research participants, deception is exposed, gratitude is expressed, and the nature and importance of the research is emphasized. One problem with debriefing is that research participants may inform potential participants of the deceptive nature of the research. It may also foster an atmosphere of mistrust. In some cases debriefing may negate a positive research outcome, for example if participants have been falsely led to believe that they are exceptionally intelligent or creative.

Many researchers believe that the stress involved in research participation is minor compared with that experienced in everyday life, and that the ends often justify the means. A therapist investigating compliance to medical advice, for example, may expose non-compliant behaviour causing guilt and embarrassment, but the data may provide important insights which could benefit many other patients. Smith states that:

> the more important the research question and the more likely the research will shed light on that question, the more subject risk that may be tolerated in comparison to subject benefits. (1975:15)

Exploitation

The relationship between the researcher and the research participants is usually an unequal one, with the researcher having more power and more knowledge of the research procedures and how the research will eventually be used. Researchers are therefore in a position to exploit research participants in ways which may be so subtle that they are barely conscious. Researchers may, for example, unwittingly make it difficult for people to refuse to participate in the study, or embarrassing for them to withdraw. They may offer incentives which people find hard to refuse, or appeal to them to 'further science', 'benefit others' or 'help me through this project'! Research participants may also comply because they mistakenly view the researcher as an important person who has the power to bring about favourable changes to their situation. Researchers must be explicit in negating this misperception.

Research participants may give up a great deal of their time, yet the researcher gets all the reward in terms of prestige, qualifications and career advancement. Participants usually enjoy their role, but unless they are treated fairly and with respect the relationship can be said to be exploitative. Researchers must avoid exploiting research participants purely for the purpose of career advancement or other personal gain.

Vulnerable people are particularly likely to be exploited; such people include those who are mentally ill or have learning difficulties. An ethical dilemma always arises when permission to involve people as research participants is granted by someone in authority, especially when the participants are in an institution or are, in some other way, 'captive'. People in this situation should make as informed a choice as possible and their rights should be carefully safeguarded. The question 'Who does the research benefit?' should always be asked.

Reporting and disseminating research findings

Ethical dilemmas are no less prevalent at the stage of reporting and disseminating research findings. Omitting information, falsifying data, and outright fraud among both professional researchers and students, usually caused by pressures to succeed, are well documented in the literature (Diener and Crandall 1978, Broad and Wade 1982). Bailey believes that 'The highest integrity must be obtained on reporting on all phases of the study exactly as they occurred' (1991:139).

This is, however, far less straightforward than it sounds. Researchers may choose to omit findings in order to protect participants or themselves, and knowledge is selected and shaped by editors and the peer review system. It is far more difficult, for example, to get research which is not statistically significant published, than that which is, leading to bias and distortion in the knowledge produced. Publishers operate with a view to the market, which can prevent the publication of certain types of knowledge while shaping and structuring that which is produced. When research is disseminated, researchers tend to lose control of it, and it may be used in ways of which they disapprove. As Rees points out:

> Facts are not inert; they can be put to a variety of purposes, malign as well as benign. Fears on this score underline the

> controversies about the inclusion of questions on racial
> background on the British decennial censuses. (1991:150)

How far researchers should be held responsible for the ways
in which their research is used is, however, a controversial
issue. Judd *et al.* state:

> there is widespread opposition to the idea that the scientist has
> any special responsibility for research utilization. According
> to this view the scientist's function is the production of
> knowledge. This knowledge is available to all and it is the
> responsibility of practical people in society to apply it.
> (1991:527)

Ideally, research findings should be made available to the
public and research participants, but whether or not it is
depends, to a large extent, on how it is disseminated. The
right to publish may be limited by sponsors, and career
advancement may induce researchers to place their work in
prestigious journals which few people read.

Research reports are often highly stylized and give the
impression that everything went according to plan.
Shakespeare and Atkinson (1993) believe that researchers
should make shortcomings in their research studies known,
and that muddle and uncertainty should be revealed and
analysed. Kimmel (1988) is of the opinion that ethical dilemmas and procedures should be written into research projects.
Rubin and Babbie are of similar mind; they state:

> In general science progresses through honesty and openness,
> and it is retarded through ego defences and deception. You
> can serve your fellow researchers – and scientific discovery as
> a whole – by telling the truth about all the pitfalls and
> problems you have experienced in a particular line of inquiry.
> (1989:55)

This is often facilitated by inviting colleagues and research
participants to assist with the task. As Anzul points out,
'Growth in self-awareness is, in itself, an ethical undertaking'
(1991:221).

Wider political issues

The research process is bound up with social and political forces of which researchers should be aware. Research findings can affect political decisions, which may be detrimental to various people in society. Research on sensitive issues such as race may increase prejudice and discrimination, or create social unrest; research aimed at producing greater efficiency in a particular industry or profession may reduce job satisfaction or give rise to widespread unemployment, and expenditure on medical research may limit expenditure on social research or social action.

Knowledge is often put to use in ways which are not beneficial to the people to whom the research is directed. Research into the treatment of a particular disease, for example, may serve to maintain the status quo by failing to address the social, economic and political factors involved in its aetiology. Similarly many disabled people are of the opinion that medically orientated research has not fundamentally altered their position (Abberley 1992, Oliver 1992). Kimmel sums up the situation thus:

> Since anything that social scientists learn can be used for ends beyond their control and even against their values, research should be undertaken only after careful consideration of its plausible consequences. (1988:117)

Tentative research findings may be applied too soon and in contexts not envisaged by the researcher; Kimmel (1988) warns against inappropriate generalization of research findings, which may be found, for example, in cross-disciplinary applied research. On the other hand, organizations may find it politically expedient to ignore research findings. The printed word has a certain mystique and researchers must be warned against the temptation of proclaiming outside their area of expertise.

Researchers hired by an organization to undertake research may be expected to work in the best interests of that organization and to 'toe the party line'. Homan gives the following example:

A researcher, 'Frank Brown' gave notice of his findings to senior members of the institutions in which he was researching; these reflected badly on their practice and they were mindful of their dependence on resources from outside, so they asked him to discontinue his research and paid him to take up another project. As his research was registered for a doctorate, this had serious personal implications . . . . (1991:131)

Offers of money from sponsors may also involve therapists in an ethical dilemma, for example they may be offered a substantial sum of money from a company involved in cigarette production, or one which supports a regime of which they disapprove. Sponsoring bodies have their own vested interests, and researchers who are dependent on them may find themselves avoiding certain research questions or methodologies for fear that their funding may be cut or withdrawn.

Government and large institutions have a monopoly on the production of knowledge as they have the resources to undertake large scale research and to utilize the findings in ways they think fit. The less powerful the group, the less influence they are able to exert.

Ethical guidelines and ethics committees

Before proceeding with a research project it is frequently necessary to submit the research proposal to an ethics committee. It is common for people to have markedly different views on ethical issues, so ethics committees typically comprise people from various professions as well as lay people. As Rubin and Babbie state, 'What is ethically "right" and "wrong" in research is ultimately a matter of what people *agree* is right or wrong' (1989:66).

Not all studies need approval by an ethics committee, and it is the responsibility of each researcher to find out what is required. This, however, is often far from clear. Owen and Davis advise, 'It is better to submit a proposal that does not, on consideration, have ethical implications, than omit to submit one that does' (1991:25). Judd *et al.* (1991) believe that as researchers are inevitably so bound up in their own research projects, they should not trust themselves to make ethical judgements without assistance. Ethics committees may highlight ethical issues which even the most discerning researchers have overlooked.

Ethics committees and ethical guidelines are not without their critics, however. Some people argue that professionals are too strongly represented on ethics committees, while others believe they are too orientated to clinical trials, with a subsequent 'black or white' approach to decision making. Plummer (1983) believes that ethical guidelines can lead to 'dogmatic sterility', and Homan states, 'ethical principles are established on the basis of a considerable measure of professional self-interest' (1991:3). He also believes that there is little consensus about ethical issues within professions.

More importantly perhaps, ethics committees tend to absolve researchers from making ethical decisions. Homan (1991) believes that they pre-empt discussion, which would be better left unfettered. Ethical values change over time and across cultures and there are no absolute right and wrong answers. The ultimate responsibility for ethically acceptable research thus lies with the researcher. As Judd *et al.* state:

> Neither the use of ethical advisers nor ethical clearance by an institutional advisory committee changes the fact that the ethical responsibility for the welfare of research participants remains with the individual investigator. (1991:484)

It is sometimes necessary, in health related research, to obtain the permission of a doctor if a researcher wishes to involve patients or clients as research participants. Similarly a doctor's consent is necessary before patients' medical records can be released. Partridge and Barnitt (1986) make the point that there is no obigation for any doctor to agree, and that his or her decision is final.

Although the rhetoric is usually in terms of protecting patients from harm, doctors may just as easily refuse access in order to protect themselves; for example they may block a study on 'patient satisfaction' if they feel it might reflect badly on their practice. The same can be said, of course, of any other person with sufficient authority to prevent a research project taking place. 'Protecting' patients, even with the best of intentions, gives rise to a further ethical question: is it right that adults who may wish to become involved in research should be denied the opportunity by other adults?

Conclusion

Researchers are frequently in a situation of conflict. They must decide whether the right to acquire knowledge overrides the right of individual research participants, whether future findings are likely to outweigh immediate costs, and whether it is better to undertake research with questionable practices than not to carry it out at all. Sim (1989) reminds us that ethical questions in research are never 'dealt with' but rather need to be constantly analysed and reappraised. Researchers can rarely be 'right' or 'wrong' when making ethical judgements, but have an obligation to be well informed. As Nachmias and Nachmias state:

> The ethical researcher is educated about ethical guidelines, thoroughly examines the costs and practical benefits of the research project, exercises judgement in each situation, and accepts responsibility for his or her choice. (1981:337)

4

Writing a Research Proposal

A research proposal is a detailed written plan of the research you intend to undertake. The term 'research proposal' is used interchangeably with 'research protocol'. You will find it necessary to write a research proposal in a number of situations; you may, for example, wish to apply for funding, clear your research ideas with an ethics committee, convince your tutors that your research plan will work, or gain the help and support of colleagues and managers. If you are applying for funding you are likely to be in competition with others, which makes it vitally important that your ideas come across as interesting, important and viable.

The people who read your research proposal will want to know exactly what your research question or hypothesis is, what purpose your research will serve, whether the methods you intend to use appear feasible, and whether you are a competent person to undertake the research. They may also require detailed plans and costings of your intended work. You will not necessarily be expected to show competence in every aspect of the research process, or to undertake the research unaided, but it is important to indicate what help and resources are available to you, such as the loan of equipment, the assistance of a statistician, and access to suitable library facilities.

Most funding bodies will provide their own forms for you to fill in. Their particular interest in your research ideas are likely to vary according to their own interests and purposes. Ethics committees, for example, will obviously be interested in the moral implications of your study, whereas charitable bodies are likely to focus on the benefit of your proposed work to their particular clients. The format your proposal will normally take is outlined below.

Title

The title should be no longer than necessary, but long enough to give an exact idea of what your proposed research is about. Make it as clear and interesting as possible; this is especially important if you are in competition with other researchers for funds.

Abstract

An abstract is a brief outline of the proposed research (usually 200 to 300 words in length) giving all the essential details of the study, including its purpose, the methods to be used, the type of analysis, and an outline of the theoretical framework wherein it fits; it is really a précis of the entire proposal. As some proposals may be accepted or discarded on the basis of the abstract, it is important to spend time making it succinct, informative and interesting. Remember too, that some members of committees who will scrutinize your proposal may not be knowledgeable of your particular subject area. Ethics committees, for example, usually include some lay members, so your proposal must be written in accessible language.

Introduction

Your introduction should 'set the scene' of your research. You will need to undertake a brief literature review to show you are familiar with work carried out in your particular field, and to fit your research ideas into a theoretical framework. You should give a clear statement of the aims of your research, the purpose of doing it, and why you think it will be useful. Partridge and Barnitt state:

> Your job is to demonstrate logically but imaginatively that there is a gap in knowledge to be filled and then to explain

how your study will contribute towards filling that gap.
(1986:37)

Methods and plan of investigation

Under this section you should give details of the methods and
procedures of data collection and analysis you intend to use.
You will also need to give some information about the
intended participants of your research, for example their age,
diagnoses, sex, and what criteria you will use to include or
exclude them from your study. The facilities and assistance
you have at your disposal should also be explained; it is
essential, however, to get confirmation of people's help in
writing before mentioning their names on your research
proposal.

It can be difficult to decide on the precise methods and
analyses to be used at such an early stage, but to do so will
help to focus and clarify your thoughts. Research is, however,
a dynamic process, and it is rarely necessary to adhere rigidly
to the information on your proposal once the research is in
progress. This will, however, depend on your funding body.

Timetable and budget

The time it will take to do the research needs careful
consideration. Research nearly always takes longer than
anticipated; if you are carrying out the research at the same
time as holding down a full-time job, and/or running a
family, your time will be limited and you will need to think
carefully about how you can fit the research into your busy
schedule. Research can also be expensive, with unexpected
costs invariably arising, so this needs careful attention too.
You may need financial assistance with stationery and postage, travel, the purchase or loan of equipment, and other
people's services or assistance. If you are planning to take
time off work to carry out the research, you will also need
money for daily living. The budget you present should be
detailed and honest with every item justified. It may be
necessary to apply to several funding bodies to secure the
resources you require.

Presenting yourself

The people who look at your research proposal will need to be assured that you are capable of carrying out the research. It is therefore wise to enclose an up to date curriculum vitae which states your qualifications, any previous research experience you have had, any articles you have had published or papers you have given at conferences, and any relevant experience which has made you particularly knowledgeable on the specific topic in question. For many areas of research, clinical experience is likely to be viewed as favourably as previous research or academic expertise.

Choosing a funding body

When funds are so hard to come by it may seem inappropriate to talk about *choosing* a funding body. Therapists cannot, however, escape the ethical issues which arise when considering the acceptance of funds from different organizations. They may, for example, dislike the idea of accepting money from certain drug companies, from charities whose views and practices do not accord with their own, or from companies with political connections of which they disapprove.

It is important that therapists are in accord with their sponsoring organizations, for researchers are in an unequal power relationship and are often compelled to comply with the ideas of their sponsors regarding the content, methods and analysis of the research. As Homan states, 'Those who offer grants for research have purposes and interests of their own . . .' (1991:29). McNeill (1990) makes the point that funds are easier to come by when policy makers are given guidance and the research is to be statistically analysed, than when it is purely academic or more qualitative in nature. Bryman (1988) points out that researchers who favour a qualitative approach often have to display 'an aura of scientific method' in order to secure funding.

Sources of funding

It is advisable for therapists, in the first instance, to approach their professional organizations for advice regarding funding for their research. Sources of funding include government (for example the National Health Service), research councils (for example the Medical Research Council), charitable trusts and foundations (for example the Joseph Rowntree Foundation and the King Edward's Hospital Fund for London), industry, and fellowships and studentships (for example those given on an occasional basis by the Chest, Heart and Stroke Association).

Conclusion

Research proposals are not easy to write, as the process forces researchers to think in detail about their research at a very early stage. It is frequently an essential exercise, however, and will do a great deal to clarify thinking and formulate plans.

5

Reviewing the Literature

The literature review is a very important part of the research process; indeed a research project may contain nothing more than a thorough and detailed literature review. Many studies, however, involve the researcher in empirical investigations where it may seem tiresome and unnecessary to look at the work of others. A literature review should, however, always be undertaken for the reasons given below:

1. It will provide you with a deep understanding of your area of interest.
2. It will suggest new ideas.
3. It will prevent you duplicating other people's research and unwittingly 're-inventing the wheel'.
4. It will help you to avoid other people's mistakes.
5. It will provide you with research results to compare with your own.
6. It will enable you to build your research on the research of others.
7. It will allow you to identify valuable measuring instruments which you can use or adapt.
8. It may help you to identify a research study which is worth repeating.
9. It may prompt you to change or modify your research questions.
10. It will help you to clarify the use of terms and define your terminology.
11. It will enable you to verify or dispute commonly held beliefs.

12. It will place your research within a context and provide it with a theoretical base.

Bailey believes that:

> a thorough review of written material on the proposed topic of study is essential if the researcher is to design a relevant, original, useful and timely research study. (1991:15)

It can be difficult to know just how much reading to do. You should certainly have a clear idea of your research question before embarking on a serious literature review, yet 'reading round' the subject and gaining breadth of information is also important. For example, if you are interested in how the parents of children with cystic fibrosis cope with their situation, it will probably be useful to consider how the parents of children with other chronic conditions cope. Similarly, because there has been relatively little research carried out on the therapy professions, it is often helpful to look at research focusing on doctors and nurses.

One thing is certain, a literature review can never be complete; there is usually far too much to read, with new pieces of information being produced all the time. There will also be endless material which is peripheral, yet relevant, to your study. None the less, there has to come a point when the reading stops and the rest of your study begins. Sommer and Sommer advise, 'When all the names and titles you encounter begin to look familiar, then you have come close to a good overview of the area' (1980:23).

A good literature review does not reveal 'all I have read' but rather critically reviews a broad selection of relevant material. Partridge and Barnitt (1986) point out that a good literature review can, in itself, be suitable for publication; indeed such review articles are invaluable to researchers when attempting to obtain a comprehensive and up to date overview in their particular area of interest.

Although the literature review will commonly be undertaken at the start of your research project, in reality it will probably become an on-going process, for as your study progresses, new ideas will emerge. Certain pieces of literature you read may also lead you in unexpected directions. As Rubin and Babbie state:

> the research review is completed at no one point in the research process. As the research design evolves, new issues requiring additional investigation of the literature will emerge. Be that as it may it is still important to initiate a thorough literature review as early as possible in the research process. (1989:83)

Sources of information

Libraries

It is important to find a library, or more than one library, that meets your particular requirements; libraries in academic institutions, such as universities, will suit the needs of many therapists. If you are a student in higher education you will have automatic access to the library, but even if you are not you may be able to gain permission to use it.

There are many specialist libraries which may be invaluable to you depending on your research topic. Examples of specialist libraries are that of the King's Fund Centre and the Royal College of Nursing. Charitable organizations such as the Royal National Institute for the Blind, the Royal National Institute for the Deaf and the Royal Association for Disability and Rehabilitation also have their own specialist libraries. These libraries may be able to provide you with up to date reference lists on your particular area of interest.

It is important to familiarize yourself with the library and to get to know the various systems in use and the facilities on offer. There is no need to struggle over this, or to feel daunted, as librarians are there specifically to help you. If you are on a course with other students, a time may be set aside during your first week to show you round the library and explain how everything works.

The library will contain various indices of authors' names, titles and subject areas. These are situated either on cards, on a computer, or on microfiche; microfiche is acetate which contains information in a minute form which is read by using a viewer which magnifies it. Whatever indexing system you use, you will find a code number alongside each reference housed in the library indicating where it is located. Computer indices will also tell you whether the book is out of the library at present and when it should be back.

Libraries also contain specialist indices; one of these is _Index Medicus_ which lists all the medical articles published in the more prestigious journals. The _Social Science Citation Index_ is a similar one for articles in the social sciences. In addition most journals provide an annual index. Lists of abstracts on various subject areas are also housed in academic libraries, either in printed form or on the computer; an abstract gives a brief description of the article to which it refers. Many articles begin with an abstract, which is invaluable to researchers in identifying relevant information.

The subject index is searched using key words. These should be very carefully selected but should not be too specific. For example, if you are interested in the topic of deafness, your key words might include 'deafness', 'hearing impairment', 'hearing disability', 'disability' and 'handicap'. If, on the other hand, your topic is 'physiotherapy', other key words might include 'therapy', 'professions allied to medicine', 'paramedical professions' and 'physical therapy'.

Another service which may be useful to you in the library is the 'on-line' computer search; this type of search needs to be undertaken with the librarian. On-line literature searches feed into broad data bases providing a wide variety of references housed in different locations in the United Kingdom and abroad. An example of a data base is Medline which contains medical references. The librarian will advise you on which data base to use.

In carrying out an on-line computer search, a number of key words, which must be carefully chosen in advance, are keyed into the computer. A list of references can then be obtained immediately, with abstracts on request. Key words are cross-referenced to enable citations to be more specific; for example, 'children' and 'disabled' may be combined to prevent the listing of articles about able-bodied children or disabled adults. It can be difficult to think of suitable key words and, if possible, it is best to sit with the librarian while the search is in progress.

Computer searches sound like the answer to every researcher's prayers but, in reality, they can be less than satisfactory, and are usually no substitute for a good manual search. The problem is that computers cannot reason, and will tend to provide all sorts of references that, while relating to the key words, are not really relevant. In addition computer searches tend to be expensive, and the data base may not contain all the references you need.

A cheap and simple way of gathering information is to consult the lists of references at the end of relevant articles and books. Those which seem interesting can then be followed up. This, in turn, will lead to other relevant material; as Sommer and Sommer state, 'Every source becomes a springboard to other sources' (1980:23). It is important to go back to the original (primary) sources rather than relying on other authors' interpretations (secondary sources). Secondary sources can be distorted, inaccurate, or placed within different contexts; the practice of depending on secondary sources excessively, where this can be avoided, is considered unscholarly.

A further service the library has to offer is inter-library loan. If your library does not store the book or article you require, it can be requested from another library. This service may be free to you, but it is not free to the library, so it is important to have a good search for the book or article before taking advantage of this service. It usually takes a few weeks to obtain material through inter-library loan, so it is important to be sufficiently organized to allow for this delay. In addition the amount of time individual borrowers can keep the book varies, but is often restricted. Unpublished theses and dissertations can also be obtained through inter-library loan.

Other sources of information

Libraries are not the only sources of information. It can be invaluable for researchers to consult individuals who are knowledgeable in their particular field of study; this has the added advantage that a useful contact for further assistance may be made. Individual authors may be contacted via the publisher, and off-prints of their articles can be obtained by writing to them directly using the address given at the end of the article. Government departments may also supply facts and figures, for example the Office of Population Censuses and Surveys, the Departments of Health and Social Security and the Department of Education and Science. Good specialist bookshops can also be invaluable.

Television and radio documentaries and attendance at conferences and meetings can also provide excellent up to date sources of information. Agencies, such as charities, are enormously helpful and knowledgeable; they are usually pleased to meet researchers to discuss their work. Researchers can also gain access to archives where documents are stored; some documents do, however, have restricted or semi-restricted access and researchers may need to enter into negotiations if they are to have a chance of viewing them (Scott 1990).

Planning your literature review

Cadbury states:

> the search for information should be well-planned and carefully organized – simply plucking likely looking titles off library shelves is not recommended as a general policy, although it can sometimes turn up surprisingly useful material. (1991:35)

Your literature search should be focused but not rigidly so; you will need to decide on your area of interest, whether you can handle articles in foreign languages, whether you are interested in research material from other countries, and whether you need to consider unpublished material, such as documents written within organizations, or academic theses. You will also need to decide how far back you want the information to go; this will depend, to some extent, on the scarcity of suitable material, which may only become apparent as your search progresses. If you come across one or two old references which are cited frequently, they are probably influential and therefore worth reading. An historical review may, of course, be an important element of your particular project, in which case you may actively seek bygone material.

Berger and Patchner (1988b) advise that if your literature search reveals little if anything in your chosen area of investigation, it can mean one of three things:

1. You have been looking in the wrong places.
2. Your research question does not make sense.
3. You have hit upon an exciting new topic which has never been researched.

With therapy research, the last explanation is a distinct possibility.

Organization

It is extremely important to organize all the material you read and gather when conducting a literature review. Compile your own index of references, ensuring that you include all the necessary information. In the case of articles, you need to record the names and initials of all the authors, the date, the title of the article, the volume and the part numbers, and the inclusive page numbers. In the case of a book you need to record the name and initials of the authors, the date, the title of the book, its edition, the publisher, and the place of publication.

If ever you quote an author verbatim, remember to record the page of the book or article from which the quotation was taken as this may be required when you come to write up your research; there is nothing more frustrating than searching for page numbers weeks or months later, especially if you have since returned the book to the library! If you are referring to a specific author in a book of readings, both the author and the editor of the book should be named. (For full information on references and how to deal with them, the reader is referred to French and Sim (1993).)

References can be stored in a card index or on a computer. It is a good idea to write a sentence or two on every article you read, even if they appear irrelevant. Some of these articles may become pertinent as your study progresses. It can also be helpful to indicate on the back of each card where the reference was obtained.

Conclusion

The literature review is an integral and important aspect of every research project, and one which is likely to continue throughout the entire process. The art of writing a good literature review is to know where to find the information, to strike a balance between specificity and generality, and to examine the information critically.

6

Sampling and Sampling Designs

> Sampling is the process whereby people (or information) are selected as being representative of a wider population. (Morison 1986:31)

A sample is a subset drawn from a given population. The population may, for example, consist of all practising occupational therapists, and the sample will consist of a small number of them. The occupational therapists are, of course, drawn from a much wider population of therapists, employees, health workers, etc., and in that sense form a sample in themselves.

From the population of occupational therapists, a smaller group may be selected from which the actual sample is drawn; this is termed the sampling frame. The occupational therapists in the sampling frame may, for example, work in a certain part of the country or in specific hospitals. In many areas of research which therapists conduct, it will be necessary to select a group of individuals, or objects such as hospitals, schools or pieces of text, from a wider population.

We are constantly sampling in our everyday lives; we may for example, look at several plants on display at the local garden centre and make the judgement that all the plants sold there are of a similar quality. We may sample the food in a newly opened restaurant and decide, after just one or two meals, that the cuisine or service is below standard. We could, of course, look at all the plants in the garden centre and try every item on the menu before making a decision, but it is unlikely that we would have the time, money or patience to do so. Mann states:

> The stall holder in the fruit and vegetable market who puts all his best tomatoes at the front of the pile and then fills the customer's bag with soft squelchy ones from the back is deliberately showing the purchaser a false sample. Practically every day in one way or another we carry out some form of sampling for ourselves in our ordinary daily round. (1985:120)

The purpose of taking a sample is often to make generalizations about the wider population. Sampling a population is obviously more practicable and convenient than attempting to survey the entire population, and it also allows the researcher to obtain high quality information from just a few people. However, Mann reminds us that:

> as soon as sampling is carried out the statements made about the cases involved become *probability* statements. Sampling must mean abandoning certainty for probability. (1985:121)

The extent to which the sample differs from the population it represents is termed the sampling error. Sampling error can never be eliminated completely, but it can be estimated statistically, allowing researchers to decide on the degree of error they are willing to accept. It is sometimes appropriate for researchers to discuss the sampling method they wish to use with a statistician.

Researchers must remember that generalization can only be made about the population from which the sample was drawn. It will be seen in later chapters that in many studies there is no intention of generalizing the findings beyond the specific sample, in which case it is immaterial whether or not the sample represents the wider population.

Sampling designs

Sample designs can be conveniently divided into two types: probability sampling designs and non-probability sampling designs.

Probability sampling designs

With probability sampling designs, samples are randomly selected and it is possible to specify the probability of each person or object being included in the sample.

Simple random sampling

With this type of sampling, sampling units are selected at random; the raffle is an example of simple random sampling. Lists are frequently obtained from which to draw the sample; these may include the electoral roll, the telephone directory, or state registers for various therapy professions. It is important to realize that even comprehensive lists such as these are unlikely to include everyone within the given population, and may not, therefore, be truly representative. Nor can people be forced to take part in research; Silverman (1977) reports that those who volunteer or eagerly return their questionnaires are rather different people from those who do not. This too can lead to samples which are less than representative.

The selection of participants is typically made by using random numbers which can often be found at the back of research methodology and statistics texts. Using random numbers has the same effect as mixing and selecting numbers from a hat, but it is more convenient. Tabulated random numbers are long, so if, for example, you are selecting 50 people, you need look only at the first two digits of each number. The numbers can be read either up, down or across, and can commence at any point; if numbers are repeated, or if they lie outside your range, for example if you come across numbers 75 or 92, you can simply ignore them and move on to the next.

Systematic sampling (quasi-random sampling)

With this type of sampling, sampling units are chosen from a list in a systematic way, for example every fifth or every twelfth person or object may be selected. McNeill (1990) makes the point that the actual number to be used in systematic sampling should be chosen randomly, as people have preferences for some numbers over others, the number seven being particularly popular.

The main problem with this type of sampling is that the numbers selected may have specific characteristics that are not always easy to identify or may bias the results. For example, every twelfth house may be at the end of the terrace, and every twentieth treatment session may fall on a Friday afternoon.

Stratified random sampling

> A stratified sample is one whose characteristics are proportionate to those present in the total population. (Sommer and Sommer 1980:187)

If a random sample is taken, there is always the possibility that it will not accurately represent the population from which it was drawn. If, for example, you take a random sample of physiotherapists from the state register, you may find that the percentage of men in your sample is higher or lower than the real percentage of male physiotherapists. Stratified random sampling avoids this occurrence by dividing the population, with regard to gender, age, race, etc., according to the particular study, and randomly selecting participants from each group. Thus stratified sampling reduces sampling error and is a precaution against freak random results.

Multi-stage sampling

With multi-stage sampling, groups are randomly sampled first and then individual participants are randomly sampled from these groups. For example, if you wanted to carry out some research on a sample of hospitalized patients with schizophrenia, you could first randomly select a group of psychiatric hospitals and then randomly select a group of patients with schizophrenia from within these hospitals. You may then go on to randomly select a further sample of patients who had been in hospital for more than 2 years, and another who had been there for less than 6 months.

This design helps to keep studies manageable and cheap by concentrating participants in a few places. If patients with schizophrenia were selected by means of simple random sampling for example, researchers would find themselves travelling all over the country.

Cluster sampling

With cluster sampling people or objects are selected in groups rather than on an individual bias. For example, groups of speech and language therapists working in specific areas of the country may be randomly selected, and then other speech and language therapists working in the same or neighbouring localities could be drawn into the sample. Like multi-stage sampling, cluster sampling saves time and expense by concentrating participants in a few regions. Mann (1985) warns, however, that if the clusters are to represent the wider population they must not differ from each other significantly, otherwise they can only be used for comparison. Homogeneity of clusters is not, however, always easy to achieve.

Non-probability sampling designs

With non-probability sampling designs the researcher's subjective judgement plays a part in the selection of the sample. These designs are less reliable than those of probability sampling, but they are generally cheaper and easier to use and may serve the needs of individual therapists very adequately, according to the nature of their projects.

Convenience sampling

With this type of sampling people or objects are selected purely for convenience; the method is thus far from random. The sample may, for example, consist of a cohort of speech and language therapy students from a particular college, a class of disabled children from a specific school, or a ward of patients from a particular hospital. Researchers using convenience samples will not be able to generalize their findings, but this may be of no importance, according to the aims of their research.

Purposive sampling (judgemental sampling)

With purposive sampling, the sample is hand picked by the researcher. For example, if the researcher has carried out a large questionnaire study, where the participants were randomly selected, he or she may then choose to interview a sample of specific people who are considered best able to answer a particular research question.

Snowball sampling

As the name suggests, with snowball sampling people who are selected are asked to put the researcher in touch with other suitable people to include in the study. It is far from random, but can be very useful if the population under consideration is unusual and difficult to trace. It can also be useful if the researcher is trying to contact everyone within a particular population.

Quota sampling

Quota sampling is the non-random equivalent of stratified sampling. An example of quota sampling is market research where the researcher stands on a street corner or in the supermarket and interviews people within particular categories according, for example, to their age, gender, race and so on. Opinion polls are commonly conducted in this way.

Quota sampling is less reliable than stratified random sampling as the people in the High Street or supermarket may not be representative of the wider population; there is also the potential for a great deal of researcher bias and error. It is, however, much cheaper and simpler for the researcher to stand in one place than to travel from house to house.

(For further information on sampling and sampling designs, the reader is referred to Henry (1990).

Which sampling method should be used?

The appropriate sampling method will depend on your research questions and the resources and time available to you. It may be vital for you to generalize your findings but, alternatively, this may not be one of your aims. In research, compromises constantly have to be made; what you want to do and what, in theoretical terms, would be best for you to do, may not be possible. For example you may ideally require a large random sample, but time and money constraints may only allow either a large convenience sample or a small random sample. In cases such as this you will need to decide whether the size or the 'randomness' of the sample is the most important factor.

What size should the sample be?

A major decision that researchers must make when planning their research is the number of participants required for their sample. The problem has no simple or general answer and will depend upon a variety of factors. Sample size should be decided in advance, otherwise it may look as if you stopped collecting data as soon as your hypothesis was supported (Sommer and Sommer 1980). With some research approaches and designs it is perfectly legitimate to have just one participant in your sample (see Chapters 10 and 14). The following factors should be taken into consideration when deciding on the size of your sample.

Practical considerations

There are many practical considerations to be taken into account concerning the availability of participants, and how much a large sample would cost in terms of time and money. Therapy students carrying out small projects as part of their final year of study, for example, would be ill advised to contemplate a sample of more than a few. It is often the case that researchers would prefer a large sample but are constrained by practical and financial factors. As noted above, some sampling designs group participants together, which can be an enormous saving in terms of time and resources.

Representation and generalization

If a representative sample is important, the sample should be large enough to provide stable values; that is, another similarly chosen sample from the same population should not yield results that diverge appreciably from those obtained. As Sommer and Sommer state, 'Other things being equal, large samples provide more reliable and representative data than small samples' (1980:189). Large samples give the principle of 'randomization' a chance to operate and the statistics calculated from them are more accurate than those from small samples (Nachmias and Nachmias 1981).

Although a small sample is subject to more sampling error, Smith believes it is less prone than large samples to non-sampling error, for example administrative, statistical and computational errors. He states:

> a carefully designed sample survey may collect more reliable data than an entire population survey simply because certain sources of error can be controlled much more effectively when only a small number of items are to be examined. (1975:106)

Variability of results

Another consideration which needs to be made when deciding on the sample size is the degree of variability in results that can be expected on the basis of previous experience. For example, experiments involving the measurement of reaction time to a stimulus such as light require fewer participants than experiments measuring complex motor skills or attitudes, because in the former case there is far less variability from one person to another. Variability is also affected by the homogeneity of the sample; the more alike the individuals are, the less variability they will display and the smaller the sample need be.

Purpose of the research

The size of the sample will also depend on the purpose underlying the research. If it is a pilot study, for example, where the purpose may be to smooth out any problems in the research design, then using a large sample would be wasteful and unnecessary. Similarly in undergraduate research the main purpose is to demonstrate to the examiners that basic research procedures have been tackled and that learning has taken place. In this situation a large sample would be neither sensible or necessary.

Size of the population

If the size of the population under consideration is small, then a small sample may represent a large proportion of the population. If, for example, you wanted to research visually impaired physiotherapists who are currently practising in the United Kingdom, your total population would be no more than 250, so a sample of 50 would be considerable. If, on the other hand, you wanted to study female physiotherapists, where the population contains many thousands, a sample of 50 might be insufficient.

Type of participants

With any research project, participants are always lost. They may become uninterested and drop out, move, fail to turn up for interview, spoil their questionnaires or forget to send them back. It is possible for researchers who have had some experience to make reasonably accurate guesses as to the likelihood of this happening in their research. It might be expected, for example, that a sample of therapists, interested in the topic under investigation, might be more reliable than a sample drawn at random from the public. If you suspect that a large number of participants will drop out of your study, or that they may be less than dependable, it is wise to start with a larger sample than you need.

Ethical considerations

There are many ethical issues which may constrain the size of a sample. There may, for example, be slight discomfort, risk or inconvenience to participants, or the participants in the control group may be at a slight disadvantage to those in the experimental group. In some extreme cases, where research has involved the use of dangerous or unpleasant procedures, the only solution for researchers has been to become the participants themselves! (For a full discussion of ethical considerations in research, the reader is referred to Chapter 3.)

Conclusion

Therapists undertake a wide variety of research projects, some of which necessitate investigating samples of participants. The sampling design and the size of the sample need careful consideration and will be affected by constraints of time and resources. These constraints are real and can become overwhelming, but it is important that those of us engaged in research keep the aims and purposes of our studies centrally in mind, whatever decisions we make. It is all too easy for the research question to be lost as practical and technical problems threaten to engulf us.

Part Two

Research Methods and Approaches

7

Surveys. 1. The Questionnaire

The questionnaire and the interview are survey methods in which information is gathered about groups of individuals in a systematic way. A questionnaire is merely a list of questions, but its construction is quite a difficult task and one which needs considerable practice.

Questionnaires can be distributed to participants in four main ways:

1. They may be delivered by post.
2. The researcher may deliver them personally, in which case groups of individuals may complete the questionnaire in one place and at one time.
3. The researcher may go through the questions verbally with each participant. This is often referred to as a structured interview and will be considered in Chapter 8.
4. The researcher may send the questionnaires to a person in authority, for example a therapy manager, who will distribute them, collect them and send them back to the researcher. It saves considerable postage if the questionnaires can be sent in bulk, especially as stamped addressed envelopes are required for their return.

As with all research methods, you must be clear why you want to use the questionnaire. The questionnaire is very familiar to us, and can reach a large number of people relatively easily; for these reasons there is a tendency to use it inappropriately. Before deciding whether the questionnaire is really what you need, you must have a clearly formulated research question and a definite idea of the kind of information you require. If you want to learn about people's deepest thoughts on some topic, for example, an unstructured or semi-structured interview would almost certainly be more suitable. It is very important that the questionnaire is only chosen if it provides the best way of answering your particular research questions or hypotheses. As Bell states:

> You will only reach the stage of designing a questionnaire after you have done all the preliminary work on planning, consulting and deciding what you need to find out. Only then will you know whether the questionnaire is suitable for the purpose and likely to yield usable data. (1987:58)

You also need to consider who your sample will comprise; a postal questionnaire is unlikely to provide useful data from young children or from people who cannot read.

Even when you have made the decision to use a questionnaire, many other factors need to be considered before you can proceed with its design. You will need to decide on the sample size that you require, as this may influence its complexity and length. If, for example, you have a large number of participants and a limited amount of time to undertake the research, you may need to keep the questionnaire short and relatively simple. You will also need to consider how you will distribute the questionnaire, how you will analyse the data, whether or not you need to consult a statistician, how honest or secretive you want the questions to be, and whether it will be your only research method. You may even find an existing questionnaire which suits your needs, or one which you can modify. (For detail of sampling and sample size, the reader is referred to Chapter 6.)

Types of question

Questionnaire items can be divided into one of two basic types:

1. Closed questions (often referred to as closed-ended questions). These questions are structured in such a way that participants' answers are constrained.
2. Open questions (often referred to as open-ended questions). These questions allow participants to answer in their own words.

Closed question

Dichotomous questions ('Yes/No' questions)

With dichotomous questions the participant is only permitted to answer 'Yes' or 'No'. With some very factual questions that is all that is required. For example:

"Were you over the age of 25 when you commenced your occupational therapy course?" Yes . . . . No . . . .

With some 'Yes/No' questions it is wise to allow participants to indicate that they do not know the answer. For example:

"Was the hospital where you currently work built before 1920?"

Yes . . . . .
No . . . . .
Don't know . . . . .

Scaled questions

A scale represents a series of ordered steps or fixed intervals which are used as a standard of measurement. Scales provide numerical scores which can be used to compare individuals and groups. With scaled questions, participants are given a little more scope to express their views than they are with dichotomous questions, but their responses are still restrained. Scales usually comprise five points. An example may be:

"I enjoy my current employment. Please circle the number that best expresses your view."

Strongly agree	Agree	Neither agree nor disagree	Disagree	Strongly disagree
1	2	3	4	5

Rather than labelling scales according to whether participants agree or disagree, a particular concept, such as 'interest' or 'enjoyment' may be expressed throughout the scale. For example:

"How interesting do you find anatomy? Please circle the number than best expresses your view."

Very interesting	Interesting	Neither interesting nor uninteresting	Uninteresting	Very uninteresting
1	2	3	4	5

The same idea must be expressed throughout the scale or great confusion will result. For example, it is no use starting the scale with 'Very enjoyable' and ending it with 'Very uninteresting'; although this sounds obvious, it is a mistake which is frequently made. The wording of the points on the scale also need attention; it is easy for participants to discriminate between 'agree' and 'disagree', but if they are asked to discriminate between 'often' and 'frequently' their responses will be unreliable. Sometimes the scale is only labelled at either end.

Attitudes are very complex and it is usually necessary, when attempting to measure them, to present several scales relating to the same concept. For example, when attempting to measure job satisfaction, you may want to ask about pay, working conditions, promotion prospects, supervision and sense of achievement. One problem with the analysis of scales is that participants can have identical overall scores but arrive at them in different ways. Some may, for example, be dissatisfied with their pay and conditions, some with the nature of the work itself, and others with their managers. Researchers are, of course, free to study individual question-naires if they wish.

Providing several scales on a topic, rather than one global question, may also help to minimize the 'halo effect'. The halo effect refers to the tendency we have to view everything about a person we like as 'good' and everything about a person we dislike as 'bad'. Thus rather than asking clinical tutors 'How well did this student perform in your depart-ment?', or 'How capable is this student of treating patients?', it would be best to break the question down into various aspects concerned with communication, assessment skills, clinical interviewing, punctuality, etc.

Scaled questions can have more than five points, but if there are more than seven, participants tend to find discrimination difficult. Some researchers prefer to keep the number of points on the scale even, for example four points rather than five; this is because the middle point of the scale can be difficult to interpret, especially if the scale is only labelled at either end.

Circling the middle point of the scale may mean that participants have no opinion on the topic, that they do not know the answer, or that they do not want to think about the question. If there are four points on the scale participants are forced to come down on one side or the other, but they may become irritated. Having no middle point can also bias the data if participants' attitudes really do lie at the centre.

A further problem with scales is that participants are inclined to circle the same number consistently; this tendency is referred to as 'response set'. As noted above, this frequently occurs with the middle point of the scale. The extremes of the scale, on the other hand, tend to be avoided. Some researchers have advocated alternating the direction of the scales as a way of reducing response set. For example, on some scales 'Strongly agree' could be placed on the left-hand side, and on others it could be placed on the right-hand side. This procedure does, however, tend to be confusing, as well as making scoring more difficult for the researcher.

Scales do not allow for inter-relationships among the items. For example, on a job satisfaction questionnaire participants may rate 'sense of achievement' as more important than salary, but this might be reversed if their salary were doubled. There is no way that scales can take account of these inter-relationships. (For further information on the construction of scales, the reader is referred to Anastasi (1976).)

Tick lists

Another method of eliciting closed answers is to ask participants to tick items from a list. For example:

"In your view which of the following treatment modalities are effective in relieving the pain of frozen shoulder? Please tick as many items on the list as you wish."

1. *Ice*
2. *Infra-red irradiation*
3. *Ultra-sound*
4. *Short-wave diathermy*
5. *Exercise*
6. *Massage*
7. *Manipulation*
8. *Interferential therapy*

When presenting a list such as this, it is wise to include an 'other' category. This having been said, participants do not use this category very readily as they find it much easier to recognize items from a list than to bring them to mind. It is important, therefore, that your list is as exhaustive as possible. This is facilitated by wide-ranging discussions, or by carrying out a detailed literature review before designing closed questionnaire items. You may wish to limit participants to a certain number of responses; with the above example, for instance, you could ask them to tick the three modalities which they believe to be most effective in relieving the pain of frozen shoulder.

You may also ask participants to place themselves in categories. For example:

"Please indicate to which age group you belong."

18–28	. . . .
29–38	. . . .
39–48	. . . .
49–58	. . . .
59 or over	. . . .

It is important to ensure that categories do not overlap. This is a common error when categorizing age groups and can cause great confusion. For example:

18–28 . . . .
28–38 . . . .
38–49 . . . .

Participants may also be asked to indicate an amount. For example:

"Please indicate how many patients you treated today?"

0–5	. . . .
6–10	. . . .
11–15	. . . .
16–20	. . . .
20 or over	. . . .

Ranking

Another type of closed question is where participants are asked to rank items on a list. For example, if you were carrying out a study to ascertain the popularity of various items on sale in the hospital canteen, you might devise the following question:

"Please rank in order of preference the following desserts on sale in the hospital canteen. Give the item you most prefer number '1' and the item you least prefer number '8'."

Bread pudding   . . . . .
Fruit salad   . . . . .
Rice pudding   . . . . .
Yoghurt   . . . . .
Apple pie   . . . . .
Jelly   . . . . .
Ice-cream   . . . . .
Steamed pudding . . . . .

The term 'prefer' would, however, be rather confusing as some participants might love bread pudding but avoid it for fear of gaining weight. This illustrates the importance of knowing exactly what information you require; for example, if what you really want to know is which item on the list participants would prefer *to buy*, you would need to phrase the question differently.

Multiple-choice questions

Closed questions can also test participants' knowledge in a multiple-choice format. It is essential that there is only one correct answer. For example:

  "The normal pH of the blood is":

1. 7.2
2. 7.6
3. 7.8
4. 7.4

It is desirable when constructing multiple-choice questions that each alternative is approximately the same length, as participants have a tendency to choose the 'odd one out'.

Matrix questions (grid questions)

If you want to ask two or more questions at once a grid can be used. Figure 7.1 illustrates this: the researcher wants to know how long a sample of physiotherapists have worked in a variety of specialities since they qualified. Participants would be asked to place a tick in the appropriate boxes.

How long have you spent in each of these specialties since qualifying?

	<1	1–2	3–4	5–6	7–8	9–10	11–12	13–14	15–16	>16
General out-patients										
Orthopaedics										
Elderly care										
Neurology										
Surgery										
Intensive care										
Psychiatry										
Obstetrics										

Years

Figure 7.1 *Matrix question*

Open questions

Open questions allow participants to answer in their own words, the only real restraint being the amount of space provided on the questionnaire. An open question might be:

"Please explain why you chose speech and language therapy as your career."

or

"Please explain why you find it difficult to come for physiotherapy treatment regularly."

Questionnaires usually have a mixture of open and closed questions. After circling a point on a scale, for example, participants may be asked to explain their view. It is also common for questionnaires to end with an open question such as:

"Please give any other information which you feel is important."

Open questions can provide a wealth of rich information, but they are difficult to analyse. In addition participants may find it arduous to express themselves in writing, or be unprepared to give the task their time. If you find you need to ask a lot of open questions, you should seriously consider whether the interview would be more appropriate.

Filter questions

Filter questions are used to indicate whether or not the questions that follow are relevant to the participant. If they are not, the participant is directed to miss them out and proceed to another question or section of the questionnaire. An example of a filter question might be:

"Did you qualify as an occupational therapist before 1980?"

Yes . . . .   No . . . .

(If your answer to this question is 'No' please proceed to section B.)

Funnel questions

Funnel questions are a series of questions which ask for more and more detailed information on one particular topic. For example:

"What problems do you believe speech and language therapists will meet in the next decade?"
"Which of these problems do you consider to be most important?"
"Choosing just one of these problems, how do you think it could best be solved?"

Using pictures in questionnaires

Pictures or photographs can be used in questionnaires. For example, in a study to ascertain children's knowledge of back care and lifting, the therapist could present the children with pictures of 'stick people' lifting objects in various positions, and ask them to indicate which they consider 'good' and which they consider 'bad'. Similarly, the points on a scale could be presented in pictorial form (Figure 7.2).

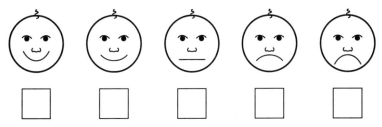

Please indicate, by ticking the appropriate box, which of the faces expresses your overall feeling about this hospital

Figure 7.2   *Pictorial question*

Wording of questions

The wording of questions on a questonnaire is vitally important and needs a great deal of care. Judd *et al.* (1991) note that even small changes in wording can bring about large changes in response. Examples of the type of question to be avoided are given below. These should be viewed merely as a guide; it can be difficult to circumvent all the problems mentioned all of the time.

Leading questions

Leading questions influence the direction of participants' replies by indicating the way in which the researcher wants them to answer. An example might be:

"Please indicate how you feel about the splendid new hydrotherapy pool."

The word 'splendid' indicates to participants that the researcher expects them to be pleased with the hydrotherapy pool.

Even if a scale is provided where shades of opinion can be expressed, the question may still be leading. For example:

"Indicate how much improvement has taken place in your pain over the last month. Please circle the point on the scale that best expresses your view."

Very much improved	Improved	No different	Is worse	Is very much worse
1	2	3	4	5

By mentioning 'improvement' in the question, the participant is given the message that this is what is expected, and that this is what the researcher wants to hear. Avoiding leading questions such as this is not always easy, though the words 'if any' after 'improvement' would make the question more neutral. One way round the problem of leading questions is to word some questions positively and other questions negatively; for example some could mention 'improvement' while others could mention 'deterioration'. This, however, tends to be confusing to participants, and to researchers when they come to analyse the data.

Leading questions can occasionally be used to advantage if the information sought involves behaviour which is socially disapproved of, leading to denial. Leading questions of this type were used by Kinsey *et al.* (1948) in their study of sexual behaviour. They have the effect of indicating to participants that such behaviour is normal and expected by researchers and that they will be tolerant of it. For example rather than asking:

"Have you taken any time off work because of your backache?"

the researcher could ask:

"How much time have you taken off work because of your backache?"

and rather than asking:

"Did you keep all your appointments?"

the researcher could ask:

"Did you keep all your appointments, or were you too busy to keep some of them?"

Smith (1975) advises that unless both alternatives are given, for example, 'coming for treatment' or 'being too busy', the question will be biased.

Rubin and Babbie (1989) point out the ethical dimension of using leading questions in this way because researchers are extracting information from participants which, under ordinary circumstances, they might not be prepared to give.

Loaded questions

Oppenheim describes a loaded question as 'one which is emotionally coloured and suggests an automatic feeling of approval or disapproval' (1966:59). Questions and statements coloured with moral judgements and evaluations should generally be avoided, otherwise the participant is likely to react to the emotional, rather than the factual, content of the question. Emotional words such as 'justice' and 'equality' should generally be avoided, as well as any word or phrase which implies the researcher's values. It is not always easy to avoid loaded questions, however, because what is regarded as judgemental by one person may be viewed as neutral by another.

People have a tendency to present themselves in the best possible light to others; this has been termed the 'social desirability' effect. This tendency operates when people fill in questionnaires, even though the questionnaire is anonymous and they will never meet the researcher. The social desirability effect is most likely to operate if participants think they might be asked to give an interview. In some questionnaires, for example Eysenk's Personality Questionnaire, a series of questions, often called a lie scale, are included as a way of detecting the social desirability effect. Such questions might include:

"Have you ever been late for work?"   Yes . . .   No . . .
"Have you ever been unkind to anyone?" Yes . . .   No . . .
"Have you ever stolen anything, even a piece of paper or a paper clip?"

                                         Yes . . .   No . . .

Participants who consistently say 'No' to items such as these, are believed to be susceptible to the social desirability effect and their scores are adjusted to accommodate this.

A series of questions, rather than a single general question, can reduce the social desirability effect. For example, in response to the question 'Do you like children?', many participants may feel they ought to say 'Yes' because society expects this of them. However, if a series of questions or statements concerning attitudes towards children are asked, rather than a single general question, a far more complex picture is likely to emerge. Such questions or statements might include:

"It is often difficult to keep one's temper with a child. Please circle the number that best expresses your view."

Strongly agree	Agree	Neither agree nor disagree	Disagree	Strongly disagree
1	2	3	4	5

"Children can be annoying if one is feeling tired. Please circle the number that best expresses your view."

Strongly agree	Agree	Neither agree nor disagree	Disagree	Strongly disagree
1	2	3	4	5

The social desirability effect may also be reduced by projective tests which gauge participants' feelings and attitudes by indirect means. An example is the Thematic Apperception Test (TAT) where participants are asked to interpret ambiguous pictures; their attitudes and feelings are then inferred from the responses they make. Another indirect method of gathering information on questionnaires is the sentence completion task, in which participants are asked to complete sentences such as 'I chose occupational therapy as my profession because . . .'. Participants' attitudes can also be inferred by asking them what *other* people think, rather than what *they* think. For example:

"What do most of your colleagues think about patients who are reluctant to be discharged?"

Covert questions such as these, as well as issues of anonymity and confidentiality, give rise to many ethical issues, which always need careful thought. (For a full discussion of ethical issues in research the reader is referred to Chapter 3.)

Multiple questions (double-barrelled questions)

These questions require more than one response and are therefore difficult or impossible to answer correctly, especially if they are closed. An example might be:

"Please indicate how much pain and stiffness you are now experiencing in your elbow."

A great deal . . . . .
Some   . . . . .
A little   . . . . .
None   . . . . .

These questions are obviously highly perplexing to participants and will create unreliable data. They will also be very confusing to researchers when they come to analyse the questionnaires.

Ambiguous questions

Ambiguous questions are ones which invite various inter-pretations; they must be avoided, especially as there is no opportunity of clarifying their meaning, as there might be in an interview. Very often the ambiguity centres around an ordinary word or phrase, for example 'frequently' or 'occasionally'. At other times the whole sentence may be ambiguous or confusing. For example:

"Please indicate how many times you carried out the exercises last week."

The participant may be left wondering whether the researcher means the number of times a group of exercises were carried out, or the number of times individual exercises were carried out.

Assuming questions (presuming questions)

These questions make assumptions about participants' life-styles, behaviour or attitudes. For example, questionnaires on disability might assume that people who use wheelchairs want to walk, or that blind people want to be totally independent. Similarly, questions such as 'Do you have adequate study leave?' or 'How can the library be improved?' assume that study leave and libraries are valued by participants.

Irrelevant questions

It is tempting to include items on questionnaires merely to satisfy curiosity, or because the information *might* be impor-tant. Irrelevant questions should, however, be avoided; they make the questionnaire longer, which may lower the return rate, and they give participants and researchers unnecessary work. In addition, if an irrelevant question irritates or offends participants, co-operation may be lost unnecessarily.

Highbrow questions

Cohen and Manion (1985) advise the avoidance of very abstract questions which use difficult or complicated language. Even if participants are known to be sophisticated people, they may not have the time or patience to deal with questions of this type. Wherever possible questions should be short and simple.

Hypothetical questions (dream questions)

Hypothetical questions ask participants to imagine what would have happened if their lives or experiences had been different. For example:

"If you won a million pounds, would you still work as a physiotherapist?"

Bell (1987) advises researchers to avoid hypothetical questions wherever possible as they rarely provide useful information and are inclined to irritate participants.

Hearsay questions

These are questions where one person is asked for the opinions or attitudes of another. For example, therapists may be asked the opinions or attitudes of disabled people. Kane advises:

> Do not ask one person the opinions or attitudes of another unless you wish to compare the first person's impressions with facts you will establish with the second person. (1985:79)

'Kitchen sink' questions

These questions, described by Kane (1985), are long and rambling, asking participants for 'everything but the kitchen sink'. An example might be:

"Please explain how you came to work here, what you think of the job, and how well it fits with your overall career plan."

'Cover the world' questions

These questions, described by Kane (1985), are complex and would probably take the participant a long time to answer; a space on a questionnaire is unlikely to be adequate. An example might be:

"How do you think the NHS will fare if the current economic climate continues over the next few years?"

Jargon-ridden questions

Questions full of jargon and abbreviations should be avoided unless you are sure participants will understand their meanings. Occupational jargon becomes so familiar to those 'in the know' that it is easy to include it unwittingly in questionnaire items.

Questions phrased in the negative

Questions phrased in the negative take longer to process cognitively, and can give rise to confusion and incorrect answers if participants are not concentrating fully. They should be avoided wherever possible. An example of a question phrased negatively is:

"Please indicate how many times you did not *do your exercises last week."*

It is much less confusing to ask participants how many times they *did* do their exercises. If negative words must be used they should be made to stand out in some way, for example by underlining them or by using bold print.

Sequence of questions

On most occasions it is best to begin the questionnaire by asking for factual information of a neutral kind. If you start with intimate or highly personal questions you may alienate the participants. Glastonbury and McKean state:

> The sequence of questions in a questionnaire warrants attention. It is worth treating this matter a bit like forming a relationship – start at a fairly easy, superficial level and gradually become more intimate and sensitive. (1991:238)

It should be noted, however, that even simple demographic questions are viewed by some participants as intimate, for example questions asking for details of age or ethnic origin. If you find you are asking a large number of sensitive questions, you should consider whether the interview might not be a better research approach. On the other hand, some participants prefer the anonymity of a questionnaire.

It is important to hold the participants' interest throughout the questionnaire, so some of the more interesting questions could be reserved until the end. It is probably best to place the more difficult or time-consuming questions in the middle of the questionnaire.

Smith (1975) suggests that 'sleeper' questions can be included to ascertain how interested participants are, by gauging their level of attention. For example, when listing the treatment modalities for relieving the pain of frozen shoulder, one or two fictitious modalities could be included. Participants who tick a large number of fictitious items such as these could then be eliminated from the study.

People like to appear consistent, so when ordering questions it is important that their answers to one question do not influence their answers to the next. This can be difficult because it is disconcerting for participants if questionnaires swing markedly from one topic to another.

Return rates

The return rate of questionnaires varies according to who the participants are, but generally speaking they tend to be low. Return rates are higher if participants complete the questionnaires under the direction of the researcher. Postal questionnaire surveys, in particular, tend to yield disappointingly low returns.

If your response rate is unsatisfactory, you should send reminders to those who failed to respond; in order to do this you must identify each questionnaire with a number before it is sent. This gives rise to an ethical dilemma regarding anonymity. A way round it is to ask participants to provide their own numbers. It is not unknown for covert practices to be adopted, such as assuring participants of anonymity but identifying their questionnaires by secret codes on the stamped addressed envelopes, such as the angle of the stamps (Judd *et al.* 1991).

Even if your return rate is good, it may by worthwhile pursuing those who have failed to reply. Silverman (1977) points out that people who fail to respond are rather different from those who do, and so by persuading them to co-operate your sample will be more representative and balanced. Reminders suffer from the law of 'diminishing returns', however, with each round yielding fewer and fewer questionnaires.

As the response rate of questionnaires is typically low, everything must be done to tempt the participant to respond. Researchers may increase the response rate by ensuring that questionnaires are easy to complete, attractive and 'user friendly', and that the psychology of the participant is taken into account. Keep in mind the hard fact that most participants will not particularly want to fill in your questionnaire. The following tips should help to improve the return rate:

1. Use good quality paper. This is particularly important if the questionnaire is to pass through the post.
2. Use a clear type-face.
3. Provide sufficient space for participants to write their responses.
4. Provide very clear instructions and repeat them at each new subsection of the questionnaire. They should be put in bold print or a different type-face from the rest of the text.
5. Make sure response boxes are in correct alignment with the questions.

6. Number the pages and indicate when pages should be turned.
7. Enclose a stamped addressed envelope.
8. Offer to send an abstract of the results to the participant.
9. Thank the participant at the end of the questionnaire.
10. Clearly specify the return date and do not make it too distant, two to three weeks is reasonable.
11. Ensure confidentiality and anonymity if this is your intention.
12. Enclose an explanatory letter which states who you are and the purpose of your study. It may help to name your sponsors (if any), your qualifications, and where you are studying. It is also important to tell participants how they were selected. Write in a straightforward, courteous way, making your research sound interesting and worthwhile.
13. Material incentives are sometimes offered to participants, which may improve return rates, but most researchers cannot afford them. It may also be regarded as coercive. Incentives are always a token rather than a repayment for the participant's time and effort. They include small sums of money, gift vouchers and items such as pens or diaries.
14. Do not make the participants work unnecessarily. Try to ensure that they complete the questionnaire at a time and in a place which is most convenient to them. Always avoid December when sending out questionnaires as people tend to be busy preparing for the festive season. Do not ask participants for information they are unable to give, or which would be inconvenient for them to find. For example, it is probably unreasonable to ask a junior therapist questions about the departmental budget.
15. People do not like admitting to ignorance repeatedly, so try to avoid too many questions where they may need to.
16. Provide participants with 'bridging statements' when topics change within the questionnaire as people tend to find sudden changes of subject disconcerting. Short bridging statements such as 'The following section will ask for your opinions on clinical education' preceding each change of topic, will help to refocus participants' thoughts.

17. If filter questions are used, make sure participants can find their way around the questionnaire without difficulty.

Pilot study

Before the questionnaires are printed in large numbers and distributed, it is important to test them on a few people to iron out any remaining problems that may have been overlooked. However careful you and your tutor may have been, a few niggling problems will usually remain; for example a question may be slightly ambiguous, or a space for an open response may be too small. If you have taken care in constructing the questionnaire these problems should be few and easy to rectify.

The people in the pilot study should be as similar to the 'real' participants as possible; it is also a good idea to include people with experience of survey research. Encourage them to be critical, and to give their opinions on the length of the questionnaire, its clarity and attractiveness, any problems they encountered with specific questions, and any adverse reactions they felt. If you have difficulty finding a sample of people to take part in your research, it is probably not worth 'wasting' them on the pilot study. In this situation it is legitimate to choose people who are dissimilar, yet as similar as possible, to the survey participants.

Analysing questionnaire data

Closed questions are amenable to a numerical or statistical analysis. To analyse data numerically or statistically, every item and subitem on the questionnaire must be given a number. You may choose to pre-code your questionnaire in this way; for example a list of items may be numbered, as may the five points on a five-point scale. If you intend to code all or part of the questionnaire after it has been completed and returned, remember to give yourself generous margins.

If your data is relatively simple and not too extensive, it is quite feasible and sensible to analyse it with a hand-held calculator. You may wish to display your data as graphs, tables, charts and simple statistics, for example means, modes and percentages. (For further information on graphics and basic statistics, the reader is referred to Chapter 11.)

If you have a great deal of information, you may decide to key your data into a computer. This may also be advisable if you want to carry out a very complex analysis. There are many statistical packages available to help you. These packages vary in what they will do; the Statistical Package for the Social Sciences (SPSS), for example, is very powerful, but other more modest packages may best suit your needs; it is very important to seek advice. Precisely how you choose to analyse your data will depend on your particular research questions or hypotheses. You may find you have too much data, in which case it will be necessary for you to make decisions as to which parts to analyse. (For further information on the use of computers in research, the reader is referred to Berger and Patchner (1988a).)

Analysing open questions is generally more difficult than analysing closed questions. Basically the researcher needs to read all the responses to an open question and identify recurrent themes, a process referred to as content analysis. For example, although participants may express their ideas in many different ways, they may be covering just a few basic issues.

It is quite possible to give these themes a number and key them into the computer, along with your quantitative data, but this has several drawbacks. First, one of the major advantages of open-ended questions, that they put 'flesh on the bones' of statistical data, will be lost. Second, coding this type of information may merely serve to dilute and distort it, and third, research is usually strengthened if more than one mode of analysis is used. (For further information on content analysis, the reader is referred to Chapter 13.)

Advantages and disadvantages of questionnaires

When deciding which research method or methods to use, the researcher has much to consider, not least the many practical issues which inevitably arise. All other things being equal, however, the questionnaire can be said to have the following advantages and disadvantages.

Advantages

1. It is relatively cheap in terms of time and money.
2. A large number of individuals can be reached relatively easily and inexpensively.
3. The lack of face-to-face contact between the researcher and the participants reduces certain psychological and social influences, i.e. the questionnaire is a relatively non-reactive technique.
4. Participants have more time to think than they do in the interview, and can complete the questionnaire in their own time.

Disadvantages

1. The information gathered is rather superficial. This, however, may be exactly what the researcher requires.
2. Lack of contact between the participant and the researcher means that questions cannot be clarified or reworded.
3. Unless questionnaires are pictorial, they are unsuitable for certain people, for example young children and those who cannot read.

Conclusion

The questionnaire is a very popular and familiar research tool and one which is of immense use to researchers. A range of questions, from those which are highly structured to those which are totally open, can be devised to answer a huge variety of research questions. It is important that therapists do not view 'open' or 'closed' questions as either 'good' or 'bad' as their applicability can only be assessed in the light of the particular research project.

8

Surveys. 2. The Interview

> An interview is a face to face meeting between two or more people where an interviewer asks questions to obtain information from one or more respondents. (Feuerstein 1986:87)

Interviewing is one of the most personal of all research methods because the researcher and the research participant come into direct contact. The interview can be used as the sole research method or as one of many methods in a multi-method approach. It can also be used as a means of gathering information prior to the main research project.

Interviews can be highly structured, where they are little more than spoken questionnaires, or totally unstructured, where they resemble an ordinary conversation. Most interviews fall somewhere between these two extremes and can be placed on the following continuum:

structured . . . . .semi-structured . . . . .unstructured

The structured interview is also referred to as 'standardized', 'formal' and 'closed'; the unstructured interview as 'non-standardized', 'informal', 'open' and 'non-directive'. In this chapter the terms 'structured', 'semi-structured' and 'unstructured' will be used. Many of the issues pertaining to questionnaires in Chapter 7, for example the preparatory work involved and the wording of the questions, are very similar for the interview; the reader is strongly advised to read Chapter 7 in conjunction with this chapter.

Structured interview

In the structured interview the interviewer exercises control over the questions to be asked, the order in which they are asked, and the precise wording of the questions. The interviewer records the participants' answers on an interview schedule, which is a coding plan devised prior to the interview.

The interview schedule closely resembles a structured questionnaire, and may contain a variety of tick lists, scales and grids (*see* Chapter 7). The major difference is that participants do not have to cope with the schedule themselves, so such factors as attractiveness and ease of use are not so important. Great care must be taken over the wording of the questions to ensure they do not bias participants' answers (see Chapter 7). (For further information on structured interviewing, the reader is referred to Fowler and Mangione (1988).)

Semi-structured interview

With the semi-structured interview the interviewer knows what information is required but is free to alter the wording and ordering of the questions with individual participants. An interview schedule may be used but allowance will be made to record individual and unique responses; often the interview schedule will merely consist of a list of questions. Although the subject matter of the interview is specified, participants are given considerable freedom to express themselves as they wish. Researchers using this type of interview encourage participants to expand on their answers by probing and prompting.

Unstructured interview

With this type of interview, no pre-planned set of questions are asked. Participants are free to express themselves without being controlled or directed in any way. The interviewer can, however, raise queries and probe interesting points as they arise. The unstructured interview is commonly used in psychiatry but can be used for research, particularly at the early stages when the researcher is gathering ideas. Unstructured interviews, and to a lesser extent semi-structured interviews, depend for their success on a reasonable level of articulacy on the part of participants.

Advantages and disadvantages of the structured interview

One of the advantages of the structured interview is that it tends to be quite brief and is therefore relatively inexpensive in terms of both time and money; it is also possible for the researcher to be assisted by other interviewers, after they have received appropriate training, as every participant is asked exactly the same questions in the same order. Structured interviews are relatively easy to code and to replicate. As the wording and the order of the questions is the same in every interview, a high level of reliability is possible, though validity may be compromised. Langley (1987) states that structured interviews emphasize reliability whereas semi-structured and unstructured interviews emphasize validity.

Despite these advantages there are various limitations to the structured interview. As the questions are decided upon in advance, and researchers are required to restrict themselves to these questions, much potentially interesting material is lost. In addition, the constraints placed upon participants may result in them feeling that the researcher is not interested in them as people, but merely as research 'objects'. A further problem is that the same question wording may mean different things to different participants, with some not understanding the question at all; despite this, researchers are not able to alter the question wording, as they would be with a less structured approach.

Advantages and disadvantages of the semi-structured and unstructured interview

Unstructured and semi-structured interviews are particularly useful when exploring relatively unknown material, when gathering in-depth information, and for learning about unique experiences; it is the method used, for example, by oral historians. The information obtained is very full and rich, unique responses are captured, and researchers are free to probe and follow up interesting points as they arise. In addition, the content of each interview may be varied so that participants can give the information they are best able to provide.

The question wording and sequence may be changed to suit individual participants; it is useful, for example, to be able to alter the wording when working with young children or people with a limited grasp of the language. In addition, what is threatening to one participant, and best left until the end of the interview when rapport has been established, may be fascinating to another, who may feel frustrated if the topic is left until the end. Changing the wording and the sequence of questions may be thought to produce highly unreliable data, but, as mentioned above, the same words can mean different things to different participants, or may not be understood at all, so using the same words consistently does not ensure high reliability.

The researcher has little control over timing, so unstructured and semi-structured interviews tend to be expensive in terms of both time and money. It is also difficult to train other people to carry out the interviews as the researcher needs a very firm grasp of the subject matter in order to know which points to explore. Because of the freedom participants are given to express themselves, topic areas tend to arise in a fairly haphazard fashion, yet imposing order on them may interfere with the free and natural flow of conversation which is one of the advantages of this approach. A further problem is that coding and analysing the results is very difficult because the data is so rich and diverse that it is not readily categorized. Reliability tends to be low and interview bias is more likely to occur than in structured interviews, for example the way in which researchers phrase questions may influence the participants' answers. Categorizing the responses is also subject to bias.

Interviewers can, of course, use a variety of approaches within the same interview. When interviewing participants with cerebral palsy, for example, the therapist may require very structured, factual information regarding the treatment the participants have received, but may prefer them to express themselves freely when talking about their own perceptions and feelings concerning the treatment.

Special types of interview

Specific types of interview have been described which can be structured, semi-structured or unstructured.

Covert interview

In the covert interview the participants do not know they are being interviewed; interviewers conceal their role while assuming another, for example the role of researcher may be concealed by the role of therapist. The advantage of covert interviews is that interviewers can obtain detailed and perhaps more honest information than they would in the conventional interview, though this will depend on the roles they are adopting. For example, a therapist who wants to know more about the social lives of patients with a particular illness may decide to obtain this information by chatting to them while they are having their treatment. Similarly a therapist may interview colleagues about their experiences while training by means of staff room conversation over a period of time.

The problem of covert interviewing is that researchers must interview in a way that is appropriate to their adopted role. As a result there are likely to be many questions which cannot be asked without arousing suspicion. This method also tends to be time consuming because if researchers ask too many questions on the same topic at any one time they will appear to be behaving oddly; in addition the deception involved in covert methods tends to place researchers under considerable mental strain. Covert methods also raise various ethical dilemmas and should not be used without a great deal of thought. (For further information on ethical issues in research, the reader is referred to Chapter 3.)

Focused interview

In this type of interview participants are free to express themselves as they wish but are strictly confined to one specific topic. The interviewer probes and prompts to keep the participant to the point and to delve more and more deeply into a very narrow area. A therapist wishing to investigate patients' experiences of pain may adopt this technique. The patients would be free to express themselves but would be strictly confined to the topic of pain experience and prevented from straying into related areas such as the experience of other symptoms.

Telephone interview

Interviewing over the telephone is a relatively inexpensive method most suitable if participants are widely scattered geographically, or if a large number are being interviewed. It is probably best avoided in anything but the most structured approach. People may be unwilling to discuss personal topics over the telephone, and supplementary information, such as non-verbal communication and details of the participant's surroundings, are not available. There are also sampling problems as people without telephones cannot be included, and not everyone has their telephone number in the directory. (For further details of telephone interviewing, the reader is referred to Lavrakas (1987) and Groves *et al.* (1988).)

The group interview

Group interviews are not used very frequently but they can be useful for gathering information prior to developing a questionnaire or interview schedule. They are invaluable if time and money are short as several participants are interviewed at the same time and place. The major disadvantage of group interviews is that the dynamics of the group, for example the tendency people have to conform and the dominance of some people over others, may mean that the views expressed are not as diverse or valid as they might have been if participants were interviewed individually. (For further information on the group interview and group dynamics, the reader is referred to Stewart and Shamdasani (1990).)

Projective techniques in interviews

Projective techniques are those in which sensitive information concerning participants' feelings and attitudes are gathered in an indirect way. For example, when interviewing young children about sexual abuse, use may be made of toys, drama, music and art. Interviewers who use these techniques are usually qualified psychotherapists.

Social psychology of the interview

Interviewing competently is not easy; like any skill it must first be acquired and then improved upon with practice. Therapists carry out an enormous number of semi-structured clinical interviews in the course of their everyday work, so in theory they should be at a considerable advantage compared with other new researchers. Practised questioning techniques, however, might not necessarily be good; poor technique may have built up and become consolidated over a period of time, often proving difficult to change. If the researcher is involved in a large project, training may be provided; watching a skilled interviewer may also help. Carrying out a few trial interviews which are recorded using a video recorder enables researchers to observe their own performances; this can help them improve their technique provided helpful and constructive feedback is given.

The interview is a social situation in which participants are voluntarily giving their time to help. The researcher should arrange to conduct the interview at a time and in a place of the participant's choosing, even if this is difficult. The researcher may wish to randomize the time and the place of the interviews, or alternatively keep the time and the place constant. For example, if some participants were interviewed in the therapy department and others at home, their responses might be differentially affected by the environment. Similarly a therapist wishing to interview participants about their symptoms may need to consider the timing of the interviews as some symptoms show a characteristic pattern throughout the day which could influence the participants' replies; their symptoms may also be affected by a long journey. On the other hand, interviewing all the participants last thing on a Friday afternoon, when they feel tired and are looking forward to the weekend, may introduce unnecessary bias into the data. As researchers may be visiting research participants for the first time and usually alone, they should always ensure that their own safety is protected, and that participants do not feel intimidated or afraid by being alone with them.

Participants are more likely to co-operate if they feel the research is worthwhile and if they know something of the person conducting it. Therapists should usually tell participants of their profession, and therapy students should mention the institutions where they are studying. At all times the participants should be treated not merely as research subjects but as human beings; the purpose of the interview should be explained, giving them sufficient time to understand, and they should be told how the results will be used and when and where they will be available for inspection. Many researchers like to give participants a copy of their interview transcript to involve them more actively, and to check the validity of the data.

Participants must be assured that their responses will remain confidential and anonymous. If they are not convinced of this it is unlikely that their responses will be entirely truthful. Alternatively, the researcher may ask the participants if they require the data from their interview to remain confidential and anonymous. If participants are unusual people, it can be difficult to ensure that they are not identifiable in research reports.

Non-verbal communication

Whichever type of interview is adopted, therapists will come face to face with participants. The participants' non-verbal communication can be a useful additional source of knowledge, but it can distort verbal information as well as enhance it. Lack of facial expression or a monotonous voice, for instance, may give therapists the impression that participants are uninterested or unintelligent, which in turn will affect their own behaviour, possibly biasing the data. Silences tend to be embarrassing and often seem much longer than they really are. Researchers should remember that the subject matter of the interview is very familiar to them but may be new to participants. Taking account of participants' non-verbal communication, their appearance and surroundings without their knowledge also raises ethical dilemmas.

Researchers may influence what participants say and how they behave, not only by their verbal input, but by their non-verbal communication. A bored expression or a hint of exasperation in the voice, for example, will be readily detected by participants, possibly leading to an alteration in their behaviour. Problems such as these can be reduced with training, but there are various characteristics known to affect participants' responses which are difficult or impossible to change, such as gender, age, status and personality (Rosenthal 1976). Accent is another relatively stable characteristic by which people evaluate each other (Honey 1989).

Uniforms are another source of non-verbal communication; they give information regarding occupation and status and may also engender feelings of respect, fear or trust. They also tend to create a psychological distance between the researcher and participant. Therapists will need to consider the benefits and drawbacks of wearing a uniform to interview; this will, in part, depend on the participants and the purpose of the interview.

Physical environment

The interview should take place in an environment where privacy is assured and where neither the participant nor the researcher will be distracted. An office with a telephone or a room where people are free to come and go should be avoided.

The physical arrangement of the furniture and the distance between the researcher and participant are also important. If, for example, the researcher sits some distance from the participant and interposes a desk between them the atmosphere will tend to be rather formal, especially if they are sitting directly facing each other. A less formal arrangement can be achieved by removing the table and sitting closer, though not too close, to the participant, and at right angles rather than face to face. The effect of the seating arrangements and the general environment on the interaction between the researcher and the participant should not be underestimated. The researcher must always remember that the interview is usually an unusual interruption of everyday routine, and that participants may not be displaying their usual behaviour.

Social and psychological environment

When interviewing it is essential that the researcher appears interested in the topic, this may be easy for the first six or seven interviews but can become difficult by the nineteenth or twentieth, even though the researcher may be very committed to the topic under investigation. The interviewer must be sensitive and provide an empathic and non-judgemental atmosphere. Therapists with counselling training and experience may be at a considerable advantage as many interviewing techniques are similar to those required of the counsellor. The interview should not be allowed to drag, but nevertheless the interviewer must give the participants sufficient time to think about the questions before answering. An effort must be made not to influence participants' answers by either verbal or non-verbal behaviour.

Researchers must do everything they can to minimize the 'social desirability' effect. This refers to the tendency people have to present themselves in as favourable a light as possible. Participants may feel that various aspects of their lives will discredit them in the eyes of the researcher, for example unemployment and personal habits such as smoking or drinking. If researchers hold strong views on some issue, they need to be particularly careful not to engender this effect.

The social desirability effect has been shown to threaten the validity of research, but researchers can minimize it by paying close attention to the wording of questions and by creating a friendly and empathic environment. The relationship with participants can, however, be problematic and skill is needed to strike the right balance. As Langley advises:

> try to establish a friendly atmosphere in which the respondent will feel relaxed enough to discuss his or her views in depth; but don't get so friendly that the interview goes right off the point. (1987:27)

Ending interviews can also be difficult, especially if there has been a series with the same participants over a period of time, and if the participants found them rewarding (Ackroyd and Hughes 1981, Atkinson 1993).

Researchers should endeavour to avoid the 'halo effect'. This effect occurs when researchers allow one piece of information about the participant, for example something which is said or the environment in which the interview takes place, to colour everything else about the participant. Harvey and Smith (1977) believe that there is a tendency to make global inferences about people on the basis of very little information. There is also an underestimation of just how much people's behaviour is affected by the situation and environment they are in, especially if they experience it as strange or intimidating.

Pilot study

Before the interviews are carried out it is important to run two or three trial interviews to iron out any problems that may have been overlooked. If researchers have taken care in designing the interview schedule, these problems should not be difficult to resolve. (For further information on the pilot study, readers are referred to Chapter 7.)

Organizing the interviews

Carrying out a number of interviews, especially when they are geographically spread, requires meticulous organization. If time or money are short it is tempting to squeeze as many interviews as possible into a day, or to travel about hoping and praying that public transport will not let you down. Something is bound to go wrong, however, and it is important that you anticipate this rather than losing participants unnecessarily because you were late, or because you did not write or telephone to confirm the time and place of the interview. The interview is unlikely to be a major event in participants' lives, though it may be an unusual one, so they should always be reminded to attend. Make sure that your tape recorder is in good order, that you have some spare batteries, and that you allow yourself enough time to rest between interviews.

Analysing the data

Quantitative data

Quantitative data are analysed in the same way as that of structured questionnaires (see Chapter 7).

Qualitative data

Dealing with the data of unstructured and semi-structured interviews can be rather difficult. If the interviews were tape recorded the researcher should transcribe them from the tape into a verbatim script. This process is very time consuming; Bell (1987) estimates that it takes about 10 hours to transcribe 1 hour of tape. Transcribing is something a competent typist using a dictaphone could cope with, however, although going through the data in detail can be beneficial to the researcher in beginning to make sense of it.

　　The researcher should then read through all the transcripts very thoroughly and devise categories in which the responses can be placed; this process is termed content analysis. Deciding on the categories to be used can be problematic: too few may limit the data, reducing its validity, but too many may make categorization very difficult and reliability poor. Researchers are advised to undertake this work as quickly as possible after the interviews while the information is still fresh in their minds.

When the categories are devised, it is advisable to ask several other people to categorize at least twenty of the responses. If the level of agreement is high, 80% or more, the categories are reliable. If agreement is low, they are unreliable and need to be changed. (For further information on content analysis the reader is referred to Chapter 13.)

Direct quotations from the interviews can be used. They are often very powerful and serve to enliven the research report, especially if a great deal of quantitative data is presented. Material which is not readily categorized but is none the less interesting should not be discarded. Points made by just one or two individuals may also be very important and should be preserved and written into the report. (For further information on writing research reports, the reader is referred to Chapter 15.)

Conclusion

When compared with other methods the interview has a number of very important advantages; indeed it is often the only suitable research method available. It is more personal and enjoyable than most methods and the response rate is higher than that of the questionnaire. This is probably because talking is less of an effort than writing and most people enjoy expressing their views to an interested person. Semi-structured and unstructured interviews are ideal for gathering detailed, rich information about participants' experiences, feelings and attitudes. They enable people to put forward their own views without being constrained by the perspectives and agenda of the researcher. The validity of structured and semi-structured interviews is, however, threatened by the interaction between the researcher and the participants. These problems are not, however, unique to the interview but will apply wherever the researcher comes into direct contact with participants.

When compared with the questionnaire the interview is both time consuming and expensive and should not be used if the questionnaire will suffice.

9

The Delphi Technique

Linstone and Turoff describe the Delphi technique as:

> a method characterized for structuring a group's process so that the process is effective in allowing a group of individuals, as a whole, to deal with a complex problem. (1975)

Stewart and Shamdasani (1990) explain that the name of this technique derives from the Oracles of Delphi in ancient Greek literature who, it was claimed, could see into the future. The Delphi technique is used to gather and analyse the opinions of experts in a given field. This is achieved by sending sequential questionnaires to a selected group of people. Often used as a means of forecasting future events to circumvent problems, its strength lies in its ability to expose differing points of view.

Example of the Delphi technique

The Delphi technique will be explained by briefly decribing a study by Hitch and Murgatroyd (1983). The topic under investigation was professional communication in cancer care. The participants in the research were nurses. They were asked to fill in three questionnaires.

First questionnaire

The first questionnaire was open ended. The participants were simply asked to list problems in communication in cancer care as they perceived them. The data were then collected and collated by the researchers; 134 problems of communication were raised.

Second questionnaire

A second questionnaire was then devised, listing all the problems which had been identified in the first questionnaire. It was sent to the same participants, who were asked to tick any of the problems which they considered important. The data were collected and collated by the researchers.

Third questionnaire

The third and final questionnaire was then constructed. All the items from the second questionnaire which were ticked by at least three-quarters of the participants were listed. At this stage the researchers combined some of the items which they considered to have similar meanings, leaving just eighteen in the final questionnaire. The questionnaire was sent to the same participants who were asked why they thought each problem of communication occurred, and to suggest any solutions they might have to alleviate the problem. The data were then collected and analysed by the researchers.

Using the Delphi technique in therapy research

The Delphi technique could be used to answer a variety of research questions of interest and concern to therapists. In every case the overall format would be similar to that of Hitch and Murgatroyd's investigation, but the details of each study would be unique. There might, for example be four rather than three 'rounds' of questionnaires, and the participants would be asked to consider particular problems in different ways.

A physiotherapy tutor, for example, could use the Delphi technique to discover how clinical managers perceive the effectiveness of massage as a therapeutic treatment, and whether it should still be taught to physiotherapy students.

Using this as an example, in the first questionnaire the participants might be asked to list the benefits and drawbacks of massage, as they perceive them. Some may, for example, mention the enhancement of the placebo effect, and the benefit of physical contact, while others may believe that massage is too time consuming, and that it encourages passivity. In the second questionnaire, these views could be listed, and the participants asked to tick those which they consider to be important.

In the third and final questionnaire, all the items from the second questionnaire which were ticked by at least two-thirds of the participants could be listed. At this point the researcher may decide to combine some of the items if they are perceived to be very similar; for example, an item 'It helps patients to relax' could be combined with 'It reduces tension', and an item 'Takes too long' could be combined with 'Not cost effective'. There is a danger when combining items that meanings may be distorted, valuable information may be lost, and researcher bias may be introduced. One way of reducing this problem is to involve others, perhaps the research participants themselves, in the analysis of the data.

In the third questionnaire the participants could be asked for their opinion on each item and whether, on balance, they believe that massage should be retained in physiotherapy education and practice.

Advantages of the Delphi technique

The value of the Delphi technique is that all the research participants are provided with feedback concerning the views of others, which gives them the opportunity to take into account aspects of the problem which they may not have considered. It might be thought that this could be achieved just as effectively through group discussion, but a major advantage of the Delphi technique is that each participant has an equal voice. As Babbie explains:

> The key is that participants can contribute equally – they don't know which comment is from the boss and which is

from the mail clerk – and since no one knows what they said initially, they can change their minds without losing face. (1992:486)

When people discuss issues in a group, many psychological forces, known as group dynamics, operate to shape their responses. People have a tendency to conform to the majority view, with some being more confident and dominant than others. Groups also tend to make riskier decisions than individuals, possibly because of a diffusion of responsibility. The larger the group the less likely are some members to contribute, while others are reluctant to state a view before they have all the facts before them, in case they appear foolish later. In addition homogeneous groups tend to comprise similar individuals, leading to a restricted range of ideas, whereas heterogeneous groups tend to be antagonistic. These problems are, to some extent, avoided if the Delphi technique is used. The participants do not meet and all remain anonymous, but they have the benefit of receiving information and feedback from each other to help them develop their own views and reach decisions. The Delphi technique is also very effective in terms of time and cost. (For a full account of group dynamics, the reader is referred to Brown (1988).)

Disadvantages of the Delphi technique

One criticism levelled against the Delphi technique is its use of experts as research participants. Deciding who the 'real' experts are is never straightforward; people perceived as experts are frequently specialists whose views are sometimes blinkered, and who may form a tight-knit, homogeneous group. Linstone (1975) points out that a single person may have greater insight than all the experts put together, a fact which is amply demonstrated in the history of science. This criticism is not too worrying, however, because 'non-experts' can be used as participants without affecting the efficiency or the structure of the technique. For example, Sullivan and Brye (1983), in their study of curriculum planning, used a sample of nurses broadly representative in terms of grade and speciality, rather than relying on the views of educators.

The psychological processes which operate when people meet in a group are not altogether lacking when people are presented with questionnaires, as they are with the Delphi technique. There may, for example, still be a tendency to conform, and the 'social desirability' effect, whereby people strive to be seen in as favourable a light as possible by others, may still operate. In addition the participants' views may be affected by knowing who the other participants are, even if they are not known by name. The decisions of the participants will also be specific to the particular time and culture of which they are a part; they may for example, be influenced by the media or by current professional concerns. A further problem, which is common to all measures of attitude and opinion, is that what people say they will do rarely tallies precisely with what they actually do.

It is necessary, if the Delphi technique is to work well, that the participants are sufficiently motivated to fill in several questionnaires; it is perhaps inevitable that some participants will drop out. Another problem is preserving the momentum of the study: delays should be kept to a minimum but this is not always easy, especially when a large number of participants are involved.

Conclusion

The Delphi technique is not well known, but is well worth considering as a means of investigating certain research questions which therapists may confront. Like all research methods it has advantages and disadvantages, but for the busy therapist it can provide a way of engaging a wide range of opinion in an efficient and cost-effective manner. As Hitch and Murgatroyd state:

> It combines the virtue of the mail survey (lack of interviewer contamination, time to sit down and ponder, no travelling costs) with those of a meeting (where the whole is greater than

the parts). The Delphi technique is relatively inexpensive in terms of both time and money; it is far easier to send out questionnaires than to arrange for a large number of people to meet together several times, it can also involve more people than would be feasible in a face-to-face meeting. (1983:422)

This chapter is based upon French (1988b).

10

Experimental and Quasi-experimental Research

The experiment is the most satisfactory way researchers have of exploring causal relationships among various factors. Very often in research, and in everyday life, it is noted that two or more factors correlate, that is they are systematically related to each other; correlation does not, however, imply causation. It may be noted, for example, that scanty dressing and cold drink sales are strongly correlated, but this does not mean that one behaviour is *causing* the other. It is likely, rather, that a third factor, the temperature, is responsible for both.

The classic experiment

In the classic experiment, the researcher manipulates one variable (the independent variable), and observes changes in another variable (the dependent variable). A variable is simply a factor which varies, and the dependent variable is the factor which may vary as a result of the independent variable. Any change which is observed in the dependent variable is termed the 'experimental effect'. While manipulating the independent variable, the researcher attempts to hold all those factors which might invalidate the experiment constant. These factors are termed 'extraneous' or 'intervening' variables and may include the temperature, the noise level, and the time of day.

Research participants are randomly allocated to either an experimental group or a control group. A pre-test is then carried out where the dependent variable, for example elbow extension, is measured in all the participants. The researcher then manipulates the independent variable in the experimental group, for example a specific form of treatment may be given. At the same time the control group is given a placebo or a different form of treatment. Extraneous variables, such as the temperature of the room, the time of day, and the amount of social contact between the researcher and the participants, are held constant both within and between the groups.

The experimental and the control group are then tested again to ascertain whether the dependent variable (elbow extension) has changed. This is termed the post-test. If there is more change in the experimental group than the control group, and if that change is found to be statistically significant, then it is concluded that the independent variable brought about the change. In a double-blind experimental design, neither the research participants nor the researchers who will analyse the data know who has received the experimental treatment and who has received the placebo. If the pre-test is likely to affect the post-test, for example if the research participants may gain practice during the pre-test, then it should be omitted. In the example above, this is unlikely but it could occur, for example if memory or a specific motor skill were tested. (For a full explanation of statistical significance, the reader is referred to Chapter 11.)

A physiotherapist may randomly allocate a group of patients with Colles fractures to an experimental and a control group. The experimental group may receive heat treatment and exercises, while the control group may receive exercises only. Some weeks later the strength and mobility of hand grip in both groups of participants may be tested. If the participants in the experimental group have a stronger hand grip than the participants in the control group, and the difference is statistically significant, it may be concluded that the heat treatment combined with the exercises was more effective than the excercises alone. Marsh (1988) makes the important point that a relationship regarded as causal at one point in time, may, in the light of new information, be found to be a correlation.

Researchers who undertake experimental research define the research problem extremely precisely and formulate hypotheses. According to McNeill, a hypothesis is 'an intelligent guess about what is happening, but in a form that can be tested' (1990:150). The *null hypothesis* states that there is no difference between the experimental and the control groups, whereas the *experimental hypothesis* (alternate hypothesis) states that there is a difference. It is the task of the researcher to try to disprove the null hypothesis. (For further discussion of hypothesis testing, the reader is referred to Chapter 11.)

Bailey (1991) points out that in a true experimental design three conditions are necessary:

1. The manipulation of one or more variable.
2. Random sampling of research participants.
3. Control of extraneous variables.

Classic experimentation is associated with the biological and physical sciences and is often referred to as laboratory research. A major aim of laboratory research is that it should be precise enough to allow other researchers to replicate it. With biological and physical research it is possible to control all or most extraneous variables, and the objects of the research (chemicals, cells, molecules, etc.) are unlikely to be affected by the presence or behaviour of the experimenter, or the general environment in which the experiment takes place.

True experimental research is, however, difficult and often impossible to undertake with human beings, for both practical and ethical reasons. Speech and language therapists investigating the effect of a new treatment for stuttering, for example, may be able to control some extraneous variables, such as where and by whom the research participant is treated, but it would be considered a gross infringement of human liberty if research participants were compelled to remain in the same room for the entire duration of the research, without any stimulation or contact with the outside world, or if they were forced to undergo treatment which, in some way, caused them distress. (For further discussion of ethical issues in research, the reader is referred to Chapter 3.)

Human research participants are also affected by the researcher (experimenter effects) and by the research procedures in a way that molecules and atoms are not. Their behaviour may be influenced, for example, by the placebo effect, or the age, gender and appearance of the researcher. In addition they may feel a need to please the researcher, or to comply with his or her demands (Rosenthal 1976).

Experimental designs

Independent subjects design

In this design the participants are randomly selected either to the experimental group or the control group.

Matched subjects design

In this design participants are matched in pairs as closely as possible. One member of each pair enters the experimental group and the other member of each pair enters the control group.

Repeated measures design

With this design the same participants are measured more than once.

These three designs attempt to eliminate systematic differences between the research participants. The repeated measures design does, of course, eliminate all subject variability and is the design of choice, provided that the first measurement does not have an effect on subsequent measurements. If this is likely to be so, the matched subjects design should be chosen. Matching is not always feasible, however, in which case the independent subjects design can be used.

Factorial designs

A therapist may carry out three separate experiments, one to examine the effect of age on recovery from surgery, one to examine the effect of anxiety on recovery from surgery, and one to examine the effect of personality on recovery from surgery. These experiments may provide interesting data, but what they will lack is any knowledge of the interaction between the three independent variables (age, anxiety and personality).

In factorial designs, two or more independent variables, known as factors, are present in the same experiment, enabling researchers to examine interactions between them. It may be found, for example, that recovery is hampered if patients are both introverted *and* anxious, but that each factor in isolation is insufficient to cause the effect. Similarly, recovery may be enhanced in older people with a particular personality profile, but not in younger people with the same personality profile.

Reliability and validity

There are very many factors which threaten the reliability and validity of experiments. These include experimenter effects, unreliable instrumentation, the placebo effect, environmental influences, and sensitization of participants to research procedures. One major criticism levelled against experimental research is that it is so contrived that it lacks validity as far as real life issues are concerned. (For further discussion of reliability and validity, the reader is referred to Chapter 1.)

Ethical considerations

Sim (1989) points out that there are three main ethical dilemmas involved with randomized controlled trials:

1. Withholding new therapy from the control group.
2. Withholding standard treatment from the control group.
3. Incurring risk to the experimental group by allowing them to receive a new treatment.

Sim (1989) states that many researchers are of the view that randomized controlled trials are only acceptable if the efficiency of the two treatments is unknown. A controlled trial may mean that other beneficial treatments cannot be given as they would act as extraneous variables. There is also controversy over whether it is justifiable to involve patients in research if the benefits will only come some time in the future. It can be argued, however, that randomization is the fairest way of selecting people for experimental treatment if that treatment is in demand and if budgets are tight. However, as Sim states:

> for most subjects, the notion that their therapy is to be decided by the toss of a coin, rather than clinical judgement, is quite alien to their usual understanding of health care. (1989:242)

Quasi-experimental research

> Sometimes social researchers are not able to achieve any control at all over the research setting, and are forced to observe the world as it occurs naturally. At the other extreme they may decide that they must contrive an artificial research setting in order to exclude the operation of unwanted variables. (Marsh 1988:226)

Quasi-experimental research falls between these two extremes. Researchers undertaking quasi-experimental research manipulate the independent variable, but their control of extraneous variables and/or randomization of research participants is lacking or partial. An example of quasi-experimental research is field research, where experimentation is undertaken in natural settings.

Some quasi-experimental designs

Time-series design (Cohort design)

With the time-series design, one group of participants is investigated at one point in time, and another group of participants is investigated at another point in time. For example, a therapy tutor may examine a cohort of first year students who have been taught physiology by means of a conventional teaching method, and the following year may examine another cohort of first year students who have been taught physiology by means of an innovative teaching method. The tutor's hypothesis may be that the students who were taught by means of the innovative method will score higher marks than those taught by means of the conventional method.

If this proves to be so, the tutor may conclude that the innovative teaching method is more successful than the conventional teaching method. However, as the groups would not be randomly selected, and as extraneous variables would not be controlled, the tutor could not be certain of this. It may be the case, for example, that changes in timetabling allowed those students taught by the innovative teaching method more time to study, that the teaching staff were more enthusiastic, or that an excellent physiology text, specific to the students' needs, had just been published. Although it is likely that the two cohorts of students were similar, changes in selection policy may have widened or narrowed the pool of applicants, resulting in important differences between them.

Non-equivalent control groups

It may be possible for the researcher to find a control group which appears similar to the experimental group even though the research participants have not been randomly selected. For example, a therapist interested in testing a new treatment for patients with head injuries may be able to find a similar group of patients in another hospital, where the treatment is not being used, to serve as a control. This control group may be a good match, but it will, none the less, be a sample of convenience. (For further information on sampling, the reader is referred to Chapter 6.)

Single case experimental designs

Experimentation usually involves groups of participants, to enable generalization of the findings to be made. The problem with group experimental studies, however, is that they do not indicate whether the treatment evaluated is suitable or unsuitable for a given individual. With group designs, the improvement or deterioration of particular individuals is not taken into account; all that we have when the study is complete is a statement about the group. Some participants may have improved, others may have deteriorated, and these effects will cancel each other out when a statistical analysis is applied; indeed, the more random the group, the less useful are the findings for any particular research participant within it.

It is not uncommon for single case studies to throw doubt on everyday assumptions and to undermine assumed relationships between variables. It can even be argued that the use of a treatment, on the grounds that its effectiveness was shown by a group experiment, could be unethical or even dangerous, as it does not take account of individual needs. This having been said, the theories generated from group studies will almost certainly guide the researcher's thoughts when designing single case studies, just as studies of individual participants may lead to the application of the research findings to groups.

The single case experimental study has been slow to develop. One of the reasons for this has been the inability of researchers to distinguish it from the uncontrolled case study, which fell into disrepute in the 1950s. Hersen and Barlow (1976) suggest that the growth of behaviour therapy has led to an increase in single case methodology on a scale large enough to attract attention, and Ottenbacher (1986) notes the rise in popularity of the single case experimental method amongst therapists.

There are many single case experimental research designs which can be used, and the reader is referred to Hersen and Barlow (1976) and Ottenbacher (1986) for a detailed account. Here just two designs will be considered, the A–B–A–B design and the A–B–C–B design.

A–B–A–B design

Let us assume that the dependent variable is the patient's ability to stand up from a sitting position. The therapist must first define the problem in such a way that it can be measured, and devise a way of measuring it accurately. This may prove difficult and the therapist may decide to break the activity down into its component parts.

The next step is to take a series of measurements of this activity over a number of treatment sessions. This will give a baseline measurement with which later performances can be compared to indicate progress. Rubin and Babbie (1989) recommend 5–10 baseline measurements to give the therapist a clear picture of the patient's level of functioning; this is phase A.

The therapist will then introduce an appropriate treatment procedure for improving the patient's ability to stand from sitting; this is phase B. During this phase the therapist will take measurements of the patient's performance over a number of treatment sessions. The treatment will then be discontinued, thus returning the patient to phase A, where again his or her ability to stand from sitting will be measured on a number of occasions. Finally, the therapist will repeat the treatment, thus returning the patient to phase B.

The results can be plotted on a graph, as shown in Figure 10.1. This shows that the patient's ability to stand from sitting improved during the treatment phase and declined when the treatment was withdrawn.

Statistical analyses, suitable for single case studies, can also be applied (Hersen and Barlow 1976, Ottenbacher 1986). Their use is, however, controversial as some people believe

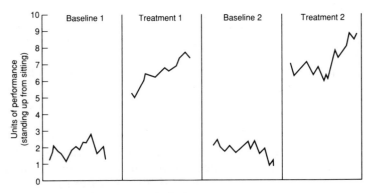

Figure 10.1   *The A–B–A–B design*

that the result is probably clinically insignificant if it is necessary to apply statistics.

One problem with the A–B–A–B design is that the improvement which results from the intervention applied in phase B may be irreversible. Once the patient has mastered the skill of standing from sitting, for example, it may be maintained despite the withdrawal of treatment. However, if the experiment is continued the therapist may find that improvement in this ability is still more rapid when treatment is given. Riddoch (1991) points out that one advantage of having a phase without treatment is that information about the natural progression of the patient's illness can be gained.

A–B–C–B design

This is a variant of the A–B–A–B design and is used to counteract the placebo effect when the treatment phase is withdrawn (Hersen and Barlow 1976). Taking an example from behaviour modification, let us imagine that the therapist is trying to stop a head-injured patient from shouting. Again, this behaviour must be defined in terms which enable measurement, and measurement devices must be devised.

During the A phase the therapist will merely record how much the patient shouts, over a period of days, in order to get a baseline measurement of this behaviour. During the B phase the therapist will intervene by offering rewards to the patient during periods of quiet, for example tokens which can be exchanged for goods in the hospital shop. The shouting behaviour is measured during this phase to ascertain whether the strategy of rewarding the patient for quiet behaviour is reducing the shouting.

If the shouting behaviour declines during the B phase, however, it can be argued that it is the result, not of the tokens, but merely of the increased attention the patient has received. Thus rather than returning to phase A, a new phase, phase C, is introduced in which the patient is rewarded with the tokens regardless of whether he or she shouts or not. After a period of time the therapist reverts to phase B in which the patient is only rewarded for not shouting.

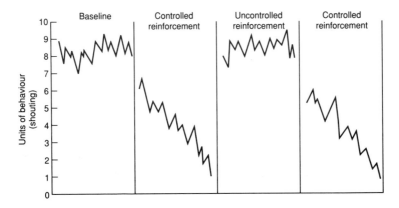

Figure 10.2   *The A–B–C–B design*

If the patient's behaviour improves most markedly during the B phases, this will indicate that reinforcing the quiet behaviour was more successful than merely paying the patient attention. If, on the other hand, the B and C phases are identical, it can be concluded that the patient's shouting behaviour declined because of the increased attention received, rather than through the positive reinforcement of quiet behaviour. Figure 10.2 illustrates the type of graph which would result if the reinforcement were successful.

Ottenbacher (1986) points out that the A–B–C–B design can also be used to evaluate alternative treatments. Going back to the example of the patient who is learning to stand up from sitting, the therapist could instigate one treatment strategy to help with this activity during phase B, and another strategy for the same activity during phase C. In this way the therapist can discover which strategy is most successful.

Advantages of single case experiments

A major advantage of single case experiments is that they integrate research with clinical practice, thereby encouraging therapists to undertake research. Single case studies can be applied flexibly, they give therapists and patients immediate feedback of the results of interventions, and have the advantage over many other methods inasmuch as the findings can be put into practice immediately. In addition single case studies may be the only feasible way of applying experimental research to patients and clients with low incidence diseases or unusual problems. Even with common conditions patients are notoriously heterogeneous, throwing doubt on the validity of many large group experiments. Single case experimental studies are also less time consuming and expensive than large scale studies.

Disadvantages of single case experiments

A major criticism of single case experiments is that they cannot be generalized beyond the individual. This, however, may be of little concern to therapists as they endeavour to assist individual patients or clients. The problem of lack of generalization can, in any event, be overcome by repeating single case studies on many individuals, that is to carry out a case series. Replication of single case studies is far more practicable than replication of large scale studies which, though advocated, is rarely carried out (Broad and Wade 1982).

Another criticism of single case experimentation is that the therapist both performs the treatment intervention and evaluates the outcome. As the therapist is so involved with both the treatment and the patient or client, it is believed that objectivity may be lacking. This problem can be overcome to some degree, however, by involving someone else in the evaluation of the treatment, at least some of the time.

Ethical issues in single case experimentation

Various ethical issues regarding single case experimentation have been identified. Faulder (1985) believes that patients should always be told that they are taking part in an experiment, but it is likely that as the single case study is so bound up with clinical practice, such considerations will be overlooked or thought unnecessary. Similarly the studies may be carried out with no consultation with ethics committees on the grounds that such tests are merely an aspect of the patient's treatment.

It can also be argued that it is ethically wrong to withhold a treatment from a patient merely for the purposes of research, and many therapists may feel uncomfortable about this aspect of single case experimentation. Therapists may worry that patients will suffer unnecessarily if treatment is withheld, that they might return to baseline measures of performance, or that they might become confused or alienated. However, Rubin and Babbie (1989) point out that there are often natural breaks in treatment programmes, for example when the patient goes home for a long weekend or when the therapist goes to a conference, and it is often regarded as good practice to withdraw treatment at various times to discover just how well the patient can cope.

Concerns about withdrawing treatment can also reflect an assumption that the treatments we give are effective and safe, neither of which may be true; the ethics of subjecting people to untested treatments can equally well be questioned. It should also be remembered that only an aspect of the treatment need be withheld. Riddoch, while acknowledging the ethical dilemmas of withholding treatment, states:

> therapists are no longer justified in claiming that a therapy has been beneficial solely because a patient reports improvement after a period of treatment. It is incumbent on therapists to demonstrate that the improvement is related to the particular therapy rather than any other factor (such as natural recovery). (1991:444)

(For further discussion of ethical issues, the reader is referred to Chapter 3.)

Conclusion

Classic experimental research is a very powerful means of establishing causal relationships. However, these designs are

frequently impossible to use with human research participants; quasi-experimental designs, where the conditions are
less stringent, are often more suitable. The single case study,
in particular, is believed by many therapists and researchers to
offer the most important way forward with regard to experimental research in clinical settings.

11

Basic Statistical Concepts

Using statistics is rather like using a tool box. Certain jobs
have to be done and in order to do them you must select from
the tool box implements which are appropriate. (Clegg
1982:6)

Many people are filled with fear and foreboding at the
thought of learning about or using statistics, probably
because of their past experience of mathematics at school.
However, although statistics is a branch of mathematics, only
very simple arithmetic is used.

In order to master statistics it is necessary to grasp the basic
principles which underlie them, and, as with any skill,
considerable practice is needed to become proficient. It is not
necessary, however, to know precisely how statistical tests
work, any more than you need to know exactly how your
washing machine or computer works. Statisticians are the
people who require a deep knowledge of statistics and they
can always be called upon for help and advice.

Levels of measurement

There are four levels of measurement which must be taken
into consideration when choosing a statistical test.

1. The nominal scale

With this scale, numbers are used merely to classify objects;
bus numbers present an example of a nominal scale. Re-

searchers would be using a nominal scale if they asked how many people or objects fell into particular categories, for example how many out patients at hospitals A and B complete their course of treatment. Just as it would not make much sense to carry out mathematical operations on bus numbers, such as adding them together and taking them away, so it is nonsensical to carry out mathematical operations on data on a nominal scale.

2. The ordinal scale

The ordinal scale involves ranking or ordering numbers. However, the numbers are not absolute and there is no guarantee that the distance between 1 and 2, for example, will be the same as the distance between 3 and 4. Five-point scales used in questionnaires are examples of ordinal scales. Adding, dividing, multiplying and subtracting data on an ordinal scale is not permitted.

3. The interval scale

The points along this scale are of equal size. Thus it is permissible to use arithmetic. The interval scale has no absolute zero point, only a man made zero point, for example 0°C. Because the zero point is not absolute, it makes sense to talk about subzero points.

4. The ratio scale

This scale is the same as the interval scale except that it has an absolute zero point. Length and weight are examples of a ratio scale. The zero point on this scale literally means 'nothing'. It would be nonsense to talk about 'minus 4 inches' (minus 10.16 cm) or 'minus 10 pounds' (minus 4.5 kg). There are a few statistical tests which require an absolute zero point.

Descriptive statistics

Most people are familiar with descriptive statistics as they are used extensively in everyday life. Descriptive statistics describe the raw data (data which has not been worked upon) of research in a way which is easily understood and assimilated. If presented with a mass of numbers, most people will not have the time or the patience to interpret them. Descriptive statistics provide a way of making the data manageable and easy to comprehend.

Measures of central tendency

The raw data of research is often converted into averages. There are three types of average, which are often referred to as measures of central tendency. These are the mean, the median and the mode.

Mean

Most people will be familiar with the mean. It is found by adding a list of numbers together and then dividing them by the number of numbers in the list. For example:

$7 + 5 + 4 + 6 + 8 = 30$
$30 \div 5 = 6.$ *Thus the mean = 6.*

The mean is useful if the numbers cluster together, as they do in the above example, but if there are any extreme scores, or the scores are widely spread, the mean can be very misleading. For example:

$3 + 1 + 2 + 4 + 65 + 5 = 80$
$80 \div 6 = 13.33.$

In this example the mean is not a typical score, it has been raised because of one extreme score in the set. It will also be noted that none of the scores in the set are the same as the mean. The mean in this example is expressed as a decimal. This often has little reality in everyday life, as in the case of the average family having 2.4 children.

Median

The median is the mid-number of a distribution of ranked numbers. For example:

7 9 24 21 22 30 32   *The median is 21.*

If there is an even number the mean of the two central scores becomes the median.

The median is a better measure of central tendency than the mean if there are extreme scores, as it is less affected by them. In the above examples, if the score of 32 changed to 132 the median would be unaffected. However, a disadvantage of the median is that if one of the central scores moves, even a little, the median changes, which makes it a very unstable measure. Ordering a large list of numbers is also a tedious procedure.

Mode

The mode is the number, in a given set of numbers, which occurs most frequently. For example:

2 3 6 20 20 20 5 2 1 4 6   *The mode is 20.*

The mode describes the typical measurement and is most useful for describing nominal data. If, for example, a student is assessed on five examinations and his or her marks are as follows:

5% 20% 55% 90% 90% 90%

then the mode of 90% will show the most typical score. Which measurement is chosen to assess the performance of this student will make an enormous difference, as the mean is 58%, the median is 72% and the mode is 90%. It may be thought fairer, in this situation, to judge the student according to the mode, especially if the low scores occurred early in the course; to use the mean, in particular, would seem harsh. The mode may, in some situations, however, misrepresent the sample as a whole. The mode of 20, in the example above, is not really typical of that set of numbers.

Other disadvantages of the mode are that it is an unstable measurement and can change if just one of the numbers in the set changes. There can also be several modes in a set of numbers, in which case they will need summarizing themselves, which reduces the use of the mode as a descriptive statistic.

It can be seen how these measures of central tendency can be used in misleading ways, tactics which are not uncommon amongst politicians and sales people.

Frequency distributions

If a group of participants are tested, it is likely that some of them will obtain the same score. The scores can be organized in a frequency distribution. For example the scores in an anatomy examination may be:

Score	Frequency
10	3
12	6
14	10
17	4
20	2

If there are a large number of research participants this type of frequency distribution would be difficult to assimilate. In this situation the frequency can be conveyed more vividly by drawing a histogram or a frequency polygon.

With the histogram the scores, or groups of scores, of the examination are placed along the horizontal axis, and the frequency at which each score, or group of scores, occurred is placed along the vertical axis. Contiguous bars are then drawn in the order of the examination scores. The frequency polygon is similar except that the frequencies of the scores are represented by dots which are joined together into a line. This is illustrated in Figure 11.1 Two or more groups can be plotted on the same, or on different, histograms and frequency polygons. It is particularly easy to superimpose several frequency polygons.

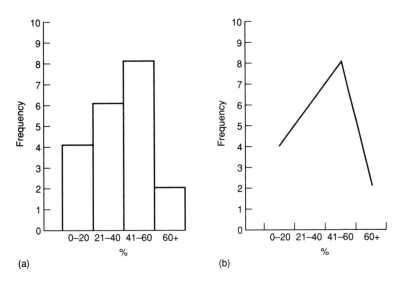

Figure 11.1 *The frequencies of various examination grades: (a) histogram; (b) frequency polygon*

Frequency polygons and histograms can only be used if the data is *continuous*, that is if it is possible and meaningful to interpolate numbers between those which are displayed. When considering examination scores this is certainly the case, but it would not be meaningful to talk about 2.5 children, or 6.2 buses, nor is it permissible to interpolate numbers after analysing data from a five-point scale. If data is not continuous it is said to be *discrete* and should be described by the use of a bar chart, which is identical to the histogram except that the bars are separated, rather than being contiguous, and can be displayed in any order.

One disadvantage of these graphs, as pointed out by Huff (1973), is that they can be used in misleading ways. The two frequency polygons shown in Figure 11.2, for example, are conveying exactly the same information, but they give a very different visual impression. Rowntree warns, 'as a consumer of statistics, act with caution; as a producer, act with integrity' (1981:190).

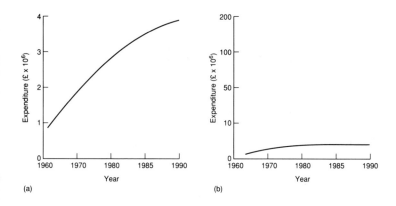

Figure 11.2 *Hospital expenditure between 1960 and 1990*

The pie chart is another way of depicting frequency. It is called a pie chart because it is cut into sections resembling the slices of a pie. Pie charts are particularly useful for describing nominal data and for comparing each category with the total. Figure 11.3 shows the percentage of patients with particular impairments at a rehabilitation centre.

Measures of variability

Measures of variability express the amount of spread or dispersion within a distribution of scores.

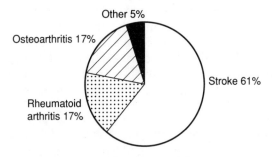

Figure 11.3 *Percentages of patients with various impairments*

Range

The range is the simplest measure of spread. It is calculated by subtracting the lowest score in a set of numbers from the highest score. For example:

2 5 6 10 14
$14 - 2 = 12$.   *The range = 12*

The range is an unstable measurement of variability because it depends on just two values, the highest and the lowest, and a change in one of these can greatly alter it.

Mean distribution

The mean distribution is a measurement which expresses how much the scores differ from the mean. To find the mean distribution, firstly the mean of a set of numbers is found. For example the mean of the set of numbers 4 6 10 4 1 is 5. The next step is to take the distance from the mean of each of the numbers in the set and add these up:

$5 - 4 = 1$
$5 - 6 = 1$
$5 - 10 = 5$
$5 - 4 = 1$
$5 - 1 = 4$

These numbers equal 12. To find the mean distribution, the mean of this number is then calculated. Thus the mean distribution is $12 \div 5 = 2.4$.

In reality, when calculating the mean distribution it is necessary to indicate whether the scores have plus or minus values when taking the distance of each score from the mean. This always adds up to 0 as the pluses and minuses cancel each other out. This can be illustrated in the example below:

$5 - 4 = +1$
$5 - 6 = -1$
$5 - 10 = -5$
$5 - 4 = +1$
$5 - 1 = \underline{+4}$
$ 0$

For these and other reasons, another very similar test of variability, the standard deviation (SD), is usually used.

Standard deviation

The standard deviation is another measurement of dispersion or spread. It is derived in a very similar way to the mean distribution by calculating the average distance of each of the scores, in a particular set of numbers, from the mean. However, to overcome the problem of the positive and negative scores cancelling each other out, these numbers are squared (when negative numbers are squared they become positive). The mean of these deviations is termed *the sum of squares*. The SD is derived by finding the square root of the sum of squares.

The larger the SD the greater the spread of a given set of scores. Thus a small SD indicates that most scores are grouped around the mean, and a large SD indicates a greater spread of scores from the mean.

When calculating the SD, information from every score is obtained, which makes it a much more stable measurement than the range.

Normal distribution

As noted above, distributions of scores are often shown by drawing graphs, termed frequency distributions, where the vertical axis indicates how often particular scores occur, and the horizontal axis represents the scores. Figure 11.4 shows

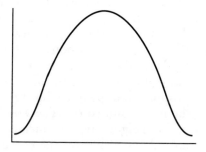

Figure 11.4 *The normal distribution*

that the normal distribution is a symmetrical, bell-shaped curve. With this distribution the mean, median and mode all have the same value. Half the scores fall above this central point and half fall below. It is a mathematical property of the normal distribution that the curve never touches the horizontal axis. Many human characteristics, such as height and weight, tend to be distributed in this way. Rowntree (1981) points out, however, that 'normal' does not imply 'usual' but rather 'idealized', 'ultimate' or 'perfect'.

If the distribution of scores is uneven it is no longer normal. If the scores fall mainly below the mean the distribution is *positively skewed.* If the scores fall mainly above the mean the distribution is *negatively skewed.* With these distributions the mean, median and mode fall at different points on the curve.

It will be seen later that some statistical tests can only be used if the data are normally, or near normally, distributed. Statistical tests are available to determine whether a set of data is normally distributed, if this is in doubt.

It is possible to specify locations on the normal curve by means of the SD. Let us imagine that a therapist has weighed a group of children and has discovered that the SD of their weight is 5 pounds (2.3 kg). Figure 11.5 represents 1 SD on the curve; that is, 1 SD covers a section of the curve. Ten pounds (4.5 kg) would represent 2 SD and 15 pounds (6.8 kg) would represent 3 SD. If the scores are normally distributed, it is always the case that 34.13% of the scores lie between the central point and 1 SD from the mean. It will be the same on both sides of the central point; thus 68.26% of the scores will be within 1 SD of the mean. In other words 68.26% of the children will deviate from the mean by no more than 5 pounds (2.3 kg). If the curve is normally distributed, 95.44% of children will lie within 2 SD of the mean, that is their weight will differ no more than 10 pounds (4.5 kg) from the mean (Figure 11.6). Thus SDs cut off fixed proportions of the normal distribution from the mean. In this example, the SD lets us know the proportion of people who are 5 or 10 pounds above or below the mean, and so on. The variable measured could, of course, be height, IQ or memory. To know precisely where an individual lies on the curve is, however, more complicated. With an SD of 5 pounds (2.3 kg) it might

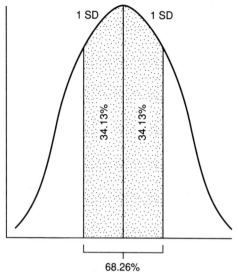

Figure 11.5   *The normal distribution representing 1 SD from the mean*

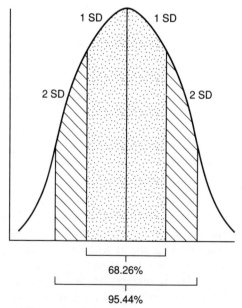

Figure 11.6   *The normal distribution representing 2 SD from the mean*

be thought that someone whose weight was 2.5 pounds (1.1 kg) above the mean would come half way between those whose weight equalled the mean and those whose weight was 1 SD (or 5 pounds) above the mean. However, because fewer and fewer people are represented under the curve as it slopes down, this is not so. To find precisely where an individual lies on the curve, a statistic called the z transformation must be carried out. (For further information on the pictorial display of data, the reader is referred to Marsh (1988).)

Inferential statistics

> inferential statistics come to our aid in helping us decide the extent to which the groups really differ. (Clegg 1982:5)

Researchers use statistics to help them decide whether research samples are similar or different. Researchers often have to make inferences about their data, and inferential statistics help them to do this; as Rowntree puts it, 'Statistics is a means of coming to conclusions in the face of uncertainty' (1981:186). For example, a therapist may try out a new treatment technique with one group of patients but keep to a tried and trusted technique with another group. It may look as though the patients receiving the new treatment are recovering faster, but this may be happening purely by chance. Inferential statistics help researchers decide whether or not this is so.

Parametric and non-parametric statistical tests

Parametric tests

Parametric tests are so called because various assumptions about the parameters of the data under consideration are made. These assumptions are as follows:

1. The sample under investigation is normally, or almost normally distributed. Statistical tests are available to determine this.

2. The scores are on an interval or ratio scale.
3. The variance of the scores in the samples under consideration are similar. Statistical tests are available to determine
this.

Parametric tests should only be used if these conditions are
met. However, slight deviations in meeting the assumptions
may not have a radical effect on the result.

Non-parametric tests

Non-parametric tests do not make assumptions about the
distribution or the variance of the data under consideration,
and can be used on data on an ordinal or nominal scale.
Non-parametric statistical tests can be used on data suitable
for parametric statistics, but they are less powerful at finding
a difference between the samples under investigation because
arithmetical operations cannot be carried out directly on the
data, so much of it is wasted.

Hypotheses

A hypothesis is a prediction. The hypothesis which the
researcher is interested in proving, for example that treatment
A will be more effective than treatment B, is termed the
experimental hypothesis (H1) or alternative hypothesis. The
above is an example of a one-tailed hypothesis because the
direction of the difference is predicted, i.e. that treatment A
will be *more* effective than treatment B. If no direction is
predicted, i.e. that treatment A will merely have a *different*
outcome to treatment B, the hypothesis is said to be two-
tailed. When looking up the result of the particular statistical
test in the tables, different values will be given for one-tailed
and two-tailed tests. The decision to use a one-tailed or a
two-tailed test must be decided *before* collecting the data.

The null hypothesis (HO) is the opposite of the experimental hypothesis, i.e. the prediction is that there will be *no*
difference between the samples. Statistical tests assume there

will be no difference, thus the researcher must strive to reject the null hypothesis.

A *type 1* error is made if the null hypothesis is rejected when it is true, and a *type 2* error is made if the null hypothesis is accepted when it is false. As the risk of making a type 1 error decreases, the risk of making a type 2 error increases, and vice versa.

Statistical significance

As noted above, inferential statistics help researchers to make judgements about how much confidence they can have in their data or, in other words, how likely it is that their results would have occurred purely by chance.

A test is said to be statistically significant if the results would have occurred by chance no more than on one occasion in twenty or, in other words, 5% of the time. After carrying out a statistical test a number will be arrived at and when this is looked up in the appropriate table, the level of statistical significance will be given. Statistical significance is expressed in terms of levels of probability, (P), the symbol $<$, (meaning 'less than'), and a decimal. Thus, if the statistical significance is $P = <0.05$, it means that the probability of the result occurring by chance is less than one in twenty. Anything above this level of chance is not statistically significant so obviously the researcher would be even more satisfied if the result reached a significance level of $P = <0.01$. or even $P = <0.001$, where the result would only have happened by chance once in a hundred or once in a thousand times respectively. Placing the minimal level of statistical significance at <0.05 is a convention and is purely arbitrary.

Statistical significance should not be confused with *real life* significance. As Rowntree (1981) points out, '"significance" does not necessarily imply "interesting" or "important"'. The level of statistical significance never tells researchers what to do, and the level of statistical significance at which they are satisfied depends upon the research topic. For example, if a new drug is being tested, a more stringent level of statistical significance than 0.05, regarding its likely side-effects, may be required before it is put into use. On the other hand, a treatment which, when tested against another treatment or no treatment at all, yields a P value of <0.1, may be clinically significant even though it is not statistically significant. If a large number of patients are benefiting from a certain treatment the therapist may be very happy to accept it, even though there is a 10% likelihood that the results are happening by chance. Conversely, a new treatment found to be statistically significant may be having a very trivial effect which is of little interest to patients.

The more often an experiment yields similar results when repeated, the more valid the findings become. Thus an experiment that repeatedly yields a P value <0.1 (which is not statistically significant), may be more significant, in the true sense of the word, than a one-off experiment which yields a highly statistically significant result. The larger the group, the easier it is to arrive at statistically significant results.

Correlation

Correlation refers to the association between two sets of scores, that is how far they 'go together'.

The data can be plotted on a graph called a scattergram, where the vertical axis expresses one of the variables and the horizontal axis expresses the other variable. If the two variables, for example IQ and examination results, are associated in such a way that an increase in one is accompanied by an increase in the other, there is a positive correlation. If, on the other hand, one variable increases while the other decreases, for example if weight increases while exercise level decreases, there is a negative correlation. Scattergrams are another example of a descriptive statistic.

When plotted on a scattergram a visual picture of the correlation is produced, as shown in Figure 11.7. Perfect positive and perfect negative correlations give straight diagonal lines, whereas if there is no correlation at all the graph is full of scattered dots. Sometimes a clear positive or negative correlation can be seen even though there is some degree of scattering. In this case the correlation is not perfect.

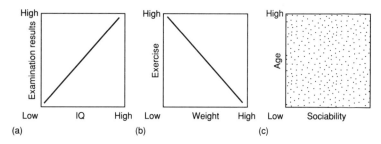

Figure 11.7   *Correlation: (a) perfect positive; (b) perfect negative; (c) no correlation*

If more detail is required concerning the strength of the correlation, and whether or not it is statistically significant, then inferential statistical tests can be applied to the data. The numbers used to express correlations are termed *correlation coefficients*. A correlation coefficient of $+1$ indicates a perfect positive correlation. A correlation coefficient of -1 indicates a perfect negative correlation. No correlation is indicated by 0.

Correlations which are less than perfect are expressed as decimals. For example, $+0.9$ expresses a strong positive correlation, and -0.2 expresses a weak negative correlation. It is interesting to note that if a correlation coefficient is squared, the resulting number represents the degree of correlation expressed as a percentage. Thus a correlation coefficient of 0.5 indicates that the variables are 25% correlated, not 50%, which is commonly believed. Tests are available to ascertain the degree of correlation among more than two variables.

Selecting a statistical test

In order to decide on the appropriate test for your data, the following questions must be asked:

1. Should a parametric or a non-parametric test be used?
2. Which test is the most powerful? The power of a test is its ability to detect a significant difference between two or

more sets of scores. Generally speaking, the test with the greatest power should be used. It is wasteful to use a non-parametric test when a parametric test could be used because non-parametric tests make less use of the data, thus increasing the risk of a type 2 error. A test can be made more powerful by increasing the size of the sample; thus a non-parametric test with 500 research participants may·be more powerful than a parametric test with 100 research participants.

3. How many samples were used in the research? Different tests are used according to whether there were one, two, or more than two samples.

4. Were the samples in the experiment independent or related? Some statistical tests are only suitable for independent subject designs, while others are only suitable for 'matched subject' or 'repeated measures' experimental designs (see Chapter 10).

Specific tests are available to analyse correlations.

Many statistics textbooks provide a useful chart which indicates which test to use.

Conclusion

In this chapter many of the basic concepts underlying statistical analysis have been discussed. Many books are available to provide greater depth of knowledge, as well as information and discussion of individual tests (see Leach 1979, Greer 1980, Francis 1988, Crawshaw and Chambers 1990, Owen and Jones 1990).

Statistical tests are useful tools for analysing certain types of research data. Some are very easy to compute and a pocket calculator is all that is required; others are more laborious, but are made easy by the use of computer packages. It is hoped that this chapter will help to demystify statistics, but for those who still feel daunted, it is a comfort to remember that statistics are only appropriate for the analysis of certain types of research data, and that it is possible to be an excellent researcher without ever using them.

Chapter

12

Observation

Observation is a research method where the researcher studies behaviour by watching and listening, either from the outside or by participating in the activities under investigation. It is suitable for investigating both verbal and non-verbal behaviour, as well as the environment in which the behaviour takes place.

Observation can be used as the main research tool, as one method among others in a multi-method approach, or as a means of gathering general data prior to the main research project. It is a very useful method for studying behaviour directly; the correlation between what people say they do, and what they actually do, is often low, which makes both the interview and the questionnaire of limited value for behavioural studies. In contrast, attitudes cannot be reliably inferred from observing behaviour.

A further benefit of observation is that research participants can be observed in their natural environment, which provides a context in which to interpret their behaviour as well as providing additional data. It is sometimes the case that people are not even aware of their behaviour until it is observed by someone else; for example, that they are interacting with women patients more than men, or that they are constantly interrupting people of lower status than themselves in meetings.

Observation requires no effort on the part of research participants, and is particularly useful for studying people who are unwilling or unable to participate in more demanding methods. Like the interview and the questionnaire, observation may be highly structured or totally unstructured, and can be placed somewhere along the following continuum: continuum:

structured . . . . *semi-structured* . . . . *unstructured*

Structured observation

In structured observation, researchers decide exactly what to observe beforehand and devise an observational schedule that will allow the information to be categorized in a highly specific and systematic way. The environment in which the observations take place may be natural or may be manipulated in some way. For example, a physiotherapist who believes that cold therapy is more effective than ultrasound in reducing traumatic swelling may test this hypothesis by observing the state of the swelling after treating one group of patients with cold therapy and another group with ultrasound over a period of time. This is an example of the experimental method which was discussed in Chapter 10. The point being made here is that observation can be an integral part of other research methods.

A highly structured approach can be used without manipulating the situation. For example an occupational therapy tutor, interested in comparing the teaching methods used on diploma and degree courses, may make very specific observations and record them in a highly structured way, but will not attempt to alter or manipulate the situation. The data obtained from structured observation is frequently suitable for statistical analysis.

Unstructured observation

In unstructured observation, researchers do not attempt to manipulate the situation they are investigating, instead they are interested in events as they occur naturally, and in the total situation rather than specific aspects of it. The data are usually recorded by means of notes, often written at the end of the day in the form of a diary. For example, a speech and language therapist interested in the interaction of clients being treated in groups could observe a number of treatment groups over a period of weeks or months. The less structured the observation, the more inferences the researcher has to make, which can lead to poor reliability and validity. On the other hand, the information gained from unstructured observation is typically far richer than that obtained from a more structured approach, which may render the data more valid. (The construction of observational schedules will be discussed later in the chapter.)

Semi-structured observation

With semi-structured observation, researchers will be more concerned with some aspects of the situation than others, but they will also be keen to record any unusual or unique events as they arise, and will give data of that type considerable emphasis in their analysis. Physiotherapists may use the semi-structured approach to observe the progress of disabled children in such activities as horse riding or swimming. Their main interest may be the children's physical development, but they are unlikely to ignore other interesting observations, such as evidence of increased sociability or improved self-confidence. With semi-structured and unstructured observation, analysis frequently takes place as the research progresses, rather than waiting until all the data has been gathered (Hammersley and Atkinson 1983).

How structured should the observation be?

Before deciding how structured or unstructured the observation should be, or indeed whether observation is the most appropriate method to use, researchers must be very clear about their research questions and hypotheses. The aims of the research must not be compromised by the use of inappropriate methods; the method should be regarded merely as a tool to enable researchers to achieve their aims.

A single observation may contain elements of the structured, semi-structured and unstructured approaches, and researchers may use different approaches at various phases of the same research project. Practical considerations must, of course, be taken into account. Observation, particularly if it is unstructured or semi-structured, tends to be very time consuming, though this will depend on the nature of each individual research project. If therapists need a free year to observe the reactions of young children to hospitalization, this will obviously be very expensive and time consuming, but if they manage to incorporate the study into their everyday work routine as paediatric therapists, then little expense will be incurred. It should be emphasized here that observing involves listening, talking and reading as well as looking; it may be perfectly in order to interview research participants and to make use of documentary evidence (see Chapter 13).

Researcher participation and participants' awareness

As well as variations in the degree of structure within observational studies, they also vary in how far researchers involve themselves in the groups they are investigating. Furthermore, the research participants may or may not be aware that they are being observed. Every observation can therefore be placed on the following two continua:

Total researcher   *No researcher*
participation . . . . *participation*
Maximum participant   *No participant*
information . . . . *information*

Thus the type of observation undertaken depends not only on the degree of structure used, but also the extent to which the researcher participates in the group, and whether or not the research participants know they are being observed.

Uncontrolled non-participant observation

This type of observation is similar to that which we all engage in much of the time. Researchers do not attempt to control the situation in any way, and the participants are not aware that they are being observed by a researcher. A researcher in this role has been referred to by Junker (1960) as a 'complete observer'.

A physiotherapist interested in the motor abilities of footballers, for example, may attend many matches as a spectator in order to observe the footballers at play. The observations may be unstructured and undertaken in order to provide ideas before embarking on a research project, or they may be highly structured where an observational schedule is used. Similarly, therapists may watch children at play through a one-way mirror to ascertain how well disabled children interact with able-bodied children; they will not be manipulating the situation in any way, and the children will be unaware of their presence.

Controlled non-participant observation

This type of observation can be seen in experimental research. Researchers remain separate from the groups they are investigating, while manipulating or controlling them in some way. For example, the staff of a centre for clients with behavioural problems may introduce various behavioural modification programmes and observe clients' behaviour to discover which are the most effective. The example given above concerning the comparison between cold therapy and ultrasound also fits this category of observation. (For further detail of experimental research, the reader is referred to Chapter 10.)

Participant observation

In participant observation, researchers are members of the groups they are investigating. As mentioned above, the extent of their participation varies, as does the knowledge that the research participants have about the researcher's presence. A term used synonymously with participant observation is ethnography (Hammersley and Atkinson 1983, Fetterman 1989), which is described by Haralambos and Holborn as 'the study of a way of life' (1990:740).

Researchers may gain access to a group and openly observe it without taking much part in its activities. For example, a therapist interested in treatment techniques used to help people with psychiatric problems could ask permission to observe other therapists at work. On the other hand, the researcher may have a secret agenda; for example, a sociologist may gain access to an occupational therapy department on the pretext that he or she is interested in taking up occupational therapy as a career, when the purpose is really to investigate professional/client communication.

It is sometimes possible to combine a genuine role with a concealed one. For example, therapists interested in the dynamics of interdisciplinary team meetings may contribute to the meetings in their role as therapists, but at the same time study the dynamics of the group in their secret role as researchers. Occasionally therapists may find themselves in an ideal situation to carry out an observational study quite accidentally. For example, a period of hospitalization may enable them to observe the behaviour of consultants, the type of interaction between patients and therapists, or the ways in which nurses organize their time.

The main advantage of honesty in observational research is that researchers are free to ask questions and to observe and record the information they receive openly. The main disadvantage is that they are likely to alter unwittingly the behaviour of the people they are observing. If a group of patients engaged in circuit training is being observed by a researcher, for example, they may try extra specially hard to succeed, making their behaviour atypical. This problem can be overcome to a large extent if researchers stay with the group for a considerable period of time, as they will then become part of the scene and people will be less affected by their presence. It can be argued, however, that provided research participants are certain of confidentiality, they may be more honest when observed and interviewed by a stranger, than by a peer or manager, because what they say and do will have no personal consequences.

Sometimes permission to carry out research may be granted by a person in authority, with those observed being forced to comply against their will. For these and other reasons, some participants may be more helpful than others, which creates the danger that researchers will rely on too few research participants for their information, leading to bias in their data; it is far easier to observe and ask questions of research participants who are friendly and co-operative than those who are not.

The complete participant

In this type of observation, which was first used by anthropologists, researchers become full members of the communities under investigation and their roles are completely concealed; for example, a person wishing to study the day to day work of physiotherapists may gain employment as a physiotherapy helper, or even go to the lengths of becoming a physiotherapist purely for research purposes. Similarly a speech and language therapist wishing to observe the activities of a self-help group may pose as a genuine member. Erving Goffman became an orderly in a psychiatric hospital to provide data for his famous book *Asylums* (Goffman 1968); Rosenhan (1980) feigned mental illness and became a patient to investigate how patients in psychiatric institutions are treated by staff; and Kirkham (1975) joined the police force as a means of studying that profession.

There are many problems with the role of participant observer, especially if the role is covert. The deception and pretence which is often involved in carrying the research through are not easy to cope with and can cause the researcher a great deal of mental strain, especially as successful observation is dependent on good co-operative relationships with the group under investigation. The researcher may come to feel great respect and friendship for people in the group and yet must continue to deceive them. It can also be argued that researchers will inevitably become so involved in the group that they will lose objectivity both when collecting and analysing the data. This problem is made worse by the fact that researchers often work alone and must usually wait until a convenient time before they can record the observations they make. If researchers' personal involvement becomes extreme, they are said to have 'gone native'. For example, a researcher who is working as a therapy helper, studying the interaction of therapists with their patients, may become so involved with the role of helper that his or her perceptions become distorted.

There are various other problems for researchers who become complete participants. First, their own behaviour may influence the activities of the groups they are investigating; therapists observing the dynamics of multi-disciplinary team meetings, for example, may consciously or unconsciously influence the proceedings of the group by their own behaviour. Second, it may be very difficult for a researcher of dissimilar background or culture to those being observed to understand their behaviour or to draw valid inferences from it, even if they are well integrated into the community. It must be said, however, that if people are observed in a natural environment over a period of time, the data often prove more valid than those obtained from a more structured approach. Third, complete participants can only study those parts of the community to which they belong. Finally, the role of complete participant can be risky; if, for example, researchers are investigating criminal behaviour, they may well get involved in illegal activities. (For further information on participant observation, the reader is referred to Jorgensen (1989).)

Junker (1960) used the following terms to describe the role of the researcher engaged in observation:

1. 'Complete observer': researchers have no involvement at all in the groups they are investigating.
2. 'Observer as participant': researchers have minimal involvement in the groups they are investigating.
3. 'Participant as observer': researchers have considerable involvement in the groups they are investigating.
4. 'Complete participant': researchers are full members of the groups they are investigating and their roles are completely concealed.

Ethical considerations

There are various ethical issues which must be examined very carefully by anyone considering the use of observation in research, especially if it is to be covert. Many groups who have been the subject of observational research, for example tramps and prisoners, have lacked the power to complain about such intrusions.

Researchers may witness events which they find disturbing, or of which they disapprove. If, for example, researchers witness the ill-treatment of clients, they will be faced with the dilemma of whether to report it or whether to continue their observations in order to document the ill-treatment later. If researchers give voice to their views they may antagonize the group they are investigating, resulting in loss of co-operation.

Many people disapprove of covert methods, so researchers must be prepared for criticism, or even worse consequences, if they publish their work. It is also possible that research of this type could be damaging to the therapy professions because, if it became widespread practice, people might become highly suspicious of therapists and would not trust them to undertake research. Others believe that covert methods can be justified if the benefits are likely to outweigh any damage that is done, or if the groups being investigated are known to be devious themselves. Considerable data on discrimination, for example, have been gathered by means of covert methods, and it is doubtful whether the data could have been collected in any other way (Fry 1986, French 1986a). (For further discussion of ethical issues, the reader is referred to Chapter 3.)

Recording and analysing observational data

Structured observation

Researchers who wish to undertake a structured or semi-structured observation will need to devise an observational schedule prior to the observation. Before doing so it can be helpful to examine schedules compiled by those who have conducted similar research. Such schedules may occasionally suffice or, more usually, may serve as a framework for the design of a new one.

Constructing observational schedules is not an easy task; each category of behaviour to be recorded must be defined very carefully; it is not enough for researchers to indicate that they will be observing 'aggression' or 'improvement' without defining what these concepts mean in terms of behaviour.

Each category must be mutually exclusive and exhaustive. This means that it should only be possible to assign each observed behavioural event to *one* category, and that it should be possible to categorize every piece of relevant behaviour observed. While devising the observation schedule, researchers should continually ask themselves whether it is a suitable tool to answer their research questions or hypotheses. If it is not, they must either change the schedule or modify it; they should never be tempted to retain a beautifully constructed schedule which does not suit their needs.

An example of an observational schedule is the Flanders's Interactional Analysis Categories (FIAC) which was devised by Flanders in 1970 (Table 12.1). It is used for observing teacher–pupil interaction in classrooms. The definition of each of these categories is given in full to guide researchers; for example, category 4 'Asks questions' is defined as 'Asking a question about content or procedure, based on teacher ideas, with the intent that a pupil will answer' (Delamont and Hamilton 1976:6). Each time an example of a given type of

Table 12.1 *Flanders's Interaction Analysis Categories*

Teacher talk	1. Accepts feeling
	2. Praises or encourages
	3. Accepts or uses ideas of pupils
	4. Asks questions
	5. Lecturing
	6. Giving directions
	7. Criticizing or justifying authority
Pupil talk	8. Pupil talk – response
	9. Pupil talk – initiation
Silence	10. Silence or confusion

behaviour occurs it is recorded on the schedule. Using this schedule, Flanders discovered that in the typical classroom in the USA, teachers talk 68% of the time, pupils 20% of the time, with 12% of the time being spent in silence or confusion (Delamont 1976).

Another example of a schedule for recording data from observations is that devised by Bales in 1950 to record the dynamics of small groups. Using this schedule, Bales discovered that groups usually contain at least one task leader, who ensures the job in hand is done, and at least one socio-emotional leader, who maintains the group process by diffusing tensions and preserving harmonious relationships. If researchers require a very detailed record of behaviour it may be possible for them to videotape the event and analyse it later. A simple observational schedule for recording the motivation of six patients is shown in Figure 12.1. It is also possible to observe and record the interaction of groups. This is illustrated in Figure 12.2.

Even with highly systematic methods of observation we always interpret what we see and hear from our own

	A	B	C	D	E	F	G	H
John	√√	√√√ √	√			√√√ √√	√√	√
Sandra	√			√		√√		√
Paul		√				√		
Lucy	√	√√√ √√√	√√		√√ √√	√	√√√ √√	√√
Derek	√√ √√	√	√√√			√√		√
Linda	√√			√	√		√√ √√	√

Categories

Figure 12.1 *A simple observational schedule*

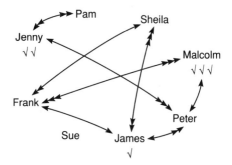

Figure 12.2 *An observational schedule showing the interaction of a group. Arrows indicate communication between individuals; ticks indicate communication with the whole group*

perspective, which can give rise to personal bias. To minimize this effect structured observations can be carried out by several researchers after a period of training. Any disagreements they have can be discussed and the schedule adjusted and refined until the level of agreement between them is high. This type of training improves reliability, but has the disadvantage that the insights of particularly sensitive researchers may be lost, with a consequent reduction of validity.

When writing the research report from structured observations it is necessary to explain the data on the observational schedule and put them into context. As Bell states, 'Useful though forms, grids and check-lists are, they cannot take account of tensions, emotions and hidden agendas' (1987:98).

Semi-structured and unstructured observation

Dealing with the data of semi-structured and unstructured observations can be rather difficult. The data is likely to be in the form of hand-written notes, often compiled after the observed events occurred. These notes may include descriptions of events, theoretical analyses, details of methods, and the researcher's own feelings and perceptions. If possible, events observed should be recorded immediately to minimize errors and distortions of memory. The use of shorthand or speed writing is always an advantage.

When the observations are complete, researchers should read through their notes very thoroughly and devise categories in which the observations can be placed. This procedure is termed content analysis. Deciding on the categories to be used can be problematic: too few may limit the data, reducing its validity, but too many may make categorization very difficult and reliability poor. (For further information on content analysis, the reader is referred to Chapter 13.)

Sampling

Deciding which situations to observe, and when and where the observations should take place, will depend on the particular research questions posed, as well as various practical considerations such as time constraints and available resources. If researchers wish to obtain representative samples of behaviour, it is better for them to observe for short periods on many occasions than to observe for long periods on a few occasions. If they wish to generalize their data beyond the particular situation they are observing, then the settings must be randomly selected. If, on the other hand, researchers want to gain a detailed understanding of the events they are observing, then it would be better for them to observe for long periods on a few occasions.

Time sampling

A systematic time sampling technique can be used to gather data. While observing a particular patient, for example, his or her behaviour could be recorded on the observational schedule every 10 seconds. Rather than being systematic, the time intervals themselves can be randomly selected.

A major disadvantage of time sampling is that important events which occur infrequently may never be observed. In addition the data tend to lack continuity; it is often unclear how events are related, especially if the time intervals between observations are long. The context in which the behaviour takes place is also partially lost. The researcher may, for example, record the aggressive behaviour of a patient being observed without fully understanding the events which precipitated it.

Event sampling

In event sampling, specific events are recorded as they occur. For example, a therapist may observe a group of elderly patients in a long stay ward to see how often they engage in certain types of behaviour, such as walking, talking to each other, or reading the newspaper. Every time the event occurs the therapist can record it. This technique is particularly useful for recording unusual or infrequent incidents; it also enables the researcher to record complete episodes from beginning to end. Time sampling and event sampling can be combined if advantages are to be gained by doing so. (For further details of sampling, the reader is referred to Chapter 6.)

Pilot study

Before an observational study is carried out it is important to undertake a few observations to iron out any problems that may have been overlooked. For example, a category may be slightly ambiguous, or an important aspect of behaviour may appear to fit nowhere on the schedule. If you have taken care in designing the observational schedule, these problems should not be difficult to solve. The people observed in the pilot study should be as similar to the 'real' research participants as possible. It is also good practice to discuss your ideas with people who have had experience of using observational research techniques themselves.

Trace measures

The use of trace measures to gather evidence is an example of unobtrusive research, which can be defined as research where little or no contact takes place between the researchers and the research participants. Trace measures are rarely used in isolation unless there is no alternative; more commonly they are employed in conjunction with other methods, such as questionnaires or interviews. They may also be used during the early stages of the research process when the researcher is attempting to generate questions or hypotheses.

Smith (1975) points out that trace measures are of two types:

1. Erosion measures – the selective wearing of surfaces and objects.
2. Accretion measures – the materials left behind by a population, for example litter, graffiti, crockery, tombstones, etc.

We are all familiar with trace measures and how they provide us with information and evidence of what is happening in our daily lives. Our suspicion may, for example, be aroused by some unexplained footprints in the garden, we may notice that the cat has taken to sleeping on the bed in our absence, or that the carpet or lawn is wearing thin in a particular place; we also judge and value the worth of objects by how well they wear. Archeologists are almost totally dependent on trace measures in their research, and the police make great use of them in their investigations, for example the analysis of DNA or fingerprints which are left behind at the scene of a crime.

Physical traces of various kinds can provide valuable data to researchers with diverse interests. The wear and tear of the grass under each item in a children's playground may give some indication of their relative use, and the degree of wear and tear on library books may indicate their popularity. Sometimes the natural setting can be manipulated a little to produce faster results; Webb *et al.* (1966) explain how the wear resistant surfaces of floor tiles can be removed to allow wear to occur at a faster rate. In this way the researcher may be able to discover the most popular items in, for example, an exhibition or an amusement arcade. Graffiti can also be used as a rich source of data for social scientists.

The effectiveness of an anti-litter campaign could be ascertained by noting the amount of litter in the vicinity of different anti-litter notices. Similarly the type of sweet wrappings found in a school playground may indicate the popularity of different items in the tuck shop, or the effectiveness of a health education programme. Sawyer (1961) estimated liquor sales by counting the number of liquor bottles in public rubbish bins.

A therapist interested in the effects of an anti-smoking campaign in the hospital where he or she works could compare the number of cigarette ends left at the end of the day, before, during and after the campaign. Similarly a therapist studying the effects of environmental change on long-stay mentally ill patients, could use measures of litter, cigarette ends and graffiti as indicators of their morale. A therapist interested in discovering which toys a group of disabled children play with most could gain some information by noting the wear and tear of the toys over a period of time, and therapists studying the gait of patients with various disabling conditions could study the wear and tear of their shoes, callipers and braces.

Advantages and limitations of trace measures in research

The main advantage of using trace measures in research is that there is no contact between the researchers and the research participants. As noted in earlier chapters, this contact can give rise to effects which threaten the validity of the research; for example, the participant may be nervous or over keen to create a good impression, and the researcher may unwittingly influence the behaviour of participants, or be unduly influenced by their accents or appearance.

Despite this important advantage, there are a number of limitations which must be borne in mind when using trace measures in research. The amount of litter or graffiti present could be highly significant but may, alternatively, merely reflect the number of cleaners employed, or the state of their morale. The researcher has little control over the situation when using trace measures, and has limited information about the population under investigation. The analysis is therefore likely to be partial, and further sources of data are usually needed before accurate interpretations can be made. Trace measures are most useful as indicators of frequency.

Temporary circumstances and seasonal variations must also be considered; the type of litter found in the school playground, for example, may reflect temporary discounts on certain items. The children may have more money to spend just after Christmas, which could influence their purchases, and the popularity of edible items may vary according to the climate. Many interpretations, other than popularity, can also be made for the wear and tear of a specific library book. It may, for example, be a set book required for an examination syllabus, or an expensive book that few people can afford to buy. Conversely a library book which is hardly touched may be so popular that everyone has gone out and bought a copy!

Conclusion

Observation is an ideal method for gathering information about behaviour. It is a relatively non-reactive method, that is, there is little contact between researchers and research participants which minimizes the effect the behaviour of each has on the other. Observation is not, of course, suitable for studying very intimate behaviour, and because of the covert nature of some observational approaches it is fraught with a greater number of ethical issues than most other research methods.

13

Documentary Research

Documentary research refers to the analysis of written documents such as official reports, textbooks, newspapers and novels, and visual and auditory material, such as films, speeches, radio and television. Pamphlets, timetables, maps, posters, notices, paintings and photography can all be used in documentary research, as well as data stored on computers.

For ease of description it is customary to divide documents into *primary* and *secondary* sources. Primary sources of data are produced by the people who gather the information or by their assistants, for example a diary kept by a researcher involved in participant observations or the transcripts of unstructured interviews. Secondary data exists before the research project begins; examples include government statistics and official reports. It is very important that secondary sources which are cited in research reports are correctly referenced, so that readers are able to find them if they wish. Scott (1990) has categorized documents into four main types:

1. Closed documents – those to which researchers have no access, such as certain government reports.
2. Semi-closed documents – those with restricted access, which may be open to researchers following negotiation.
3. Open archival documents – those which are available and are situated in archives.
4. Open published documents – those which are published and readily available in shops and libraries.

When analysing any document researchers need to ask themselves the following questions.

How representative is the document?

Existing documents are often unrepresentative of others of their type. Some documents are deliberately destroyed, and those which are housed in archives are generally selected from a far larger sample. Documents, such as letters and diaries, from as little as a century ago would only have been written by educated people, while biographies focus almost exclusively on the famous and exceptional. Which statistics are considered worthy of collection is also important; there is far more official information on poor people in our society than rich people because the former are subject to greater assessment by professionals and the state. In contrast, oppressed and minority groups, such as women, are often invisible in statistics, as though their existence is of little if any importance (Oakley and Oakley 1979). It does not necessarily matter that documents are unrepresentative, but it is vital that researchers know that this is the case in order to reach valid conclusions in their research.

Is the document authentic?

This issue is unlikely to be of great significance to therapists undertaking documentary research, but it can be vital to historians when, for example, an old document or a lost painting is discovered. It is also an issue of central concern to the police as they attempt to ascertain whether a letter is genuine or a forgery, or whether a sample of handwriting is that of a wanted criminal. For therapists the issue could become important in cases of litigation, where the authenticity of a medical record may be in doubt.

Is the document credible?

It is important that researchers discover just how accurate the document is. In order to ascertain the credibility of a document it is necessary to have some information about the author and to know why the document was written. Was it written to show the author in the best possible light? Was it for purposes of propaganda? Was it written under someone else's direction? It is also important to know whether the document is complete, and how long after the event it was produced, as memory is notoriously unreliable.

What does the document mean?

Researchers should make every effort to understand the meaning of documents. To achieve this it is necessary to comprehend the conditions under which they were produced. As Scott states, 'The particular way in which a concept was defined and applied in practice changes over time and from place to place' (1990:8). Ways of recording data vary, and are based on underlying assumptions and perceptions which are shaped by political, cultural and ideological factors. The terminology and classification of illness, for example, has changed over the years and differs from country to country; in Britain old age was classified as a cause of death until the beginning of the twentieth century, and scarlet fever and diphtheria were classified as one disease until 1855.

In a very real sense data are not *collected* but *created*. Whether or not a death is classified as suicide, for example, will depend on the ideas and perceptions of coroners at a given point in history, which will, in turn, be influenced by the society of which they are a part. Similarly, government statistics on illness reflect the biomedical concerns of western medicine (Doyal 1979). The construction of meaning is a circular process with official definitions shaping everyday definitions and vice versa. It is also a political process as certain groups have the power to impose their meanings on others. There is often little consensus, however, with agencies tending to define such concepts as 'unemployment', 'old age', 'health' and 'disability' in diverse ways. It is essential that therapists attempt to grasp the underlying meaning of any document they use in research.

It can be seen from this discussion of meaning that documents can be used for two distinct, but inter-related, purposes in research. They may be used as sources of information, for example when a therapist consults a statistical report to discover the extent of industrial accidents; or they may, of themselves, be the focus of study, for example when a therapist investigates their creation in order to understand the assumptions and perceptions underlying illness at a given time.

Content analysis

Documents are analysed by means of content analysis, which is defined by Sommer and Sommer as 'a technique for systematically describing written, spoken or visual communication' (1980:112).

When undertaking a content analysis, it is necessary to formulate the research question, and then to define and select the documents to be analysed. For example, a therapist wishing to investigate whether or not his or her profession has become more involved in research activity over the years may decide to analyse the profession's major journal to discover whether the number of research articles written by therapists has increased, and how much discussion of research exists on the letter page. It will not be possible for the therapist to analyse every journal, of course, so sampling will be necessary. Perhaps the therapist will concentrate on the last 10 years of journals and take a random sample of five from each. (For further information on sampling, the reader is referred to Chapter 6.)

Measuring the data

The data contained within documents and audio and visual material may be measured in terms of their structure and their content.

Quantity (time and space)

This may include the measurement of column inches, the size of print, or the length of a speech or radio programme. Colour and the location of items or photographs on a page can also be measured. Such measures can indicate the importance of a topic or the status of the person involved with presenting it. For example, a great many column inches in newspapers are devoted to the topic of acquired immune deficiency syndrome (AIDS) at the present time, and the length of time a person is given to make a speech can be an indication of his or her status.

Frequency

The number of times a specific item, such as a word, image or theme, occurs in a document can be counted. For example, a therapist investigating ageism in the professions might analyse the advertisement section of several professional journals or textbooks to ascertain the amount of ageist language used. The therapist may also note the number of young and elderly people depicted, and whether or not this reflects reality. Frequency counts can give an indication of underlying perceptions and assumptions, and may be a useful indicator of the importance of a topic. It can also be used to ascertain the authenticity of a document, as people are individualistic in the words and phrases they use. This type of analysis can often be performed by computer.

Intensity

This is a rather more subjective measure as it depends on the researcher making judgements. For example, a therapist analysing a report concerning disabled people may classify words or ideas as 'positive', 'neutral' or 'negative', or a therapist reading the results of various case studies concerning the effectiveness of a behaviour modification programme may classify them as 'good', 'fair' or 'poor'. Tutors marking examination scripts are also required to make judgements of this type.

Manifest and latent content

Manifest content refers to the visible, surface content of a document, whereas latent content refers to its underlying meaning. Manifest content is more objective, but latent content is often more revealing. Whether researchers concentrate on the manifest or the latent content of a document depends on their underlying research questions. Concentrating on latent content involves 'reading between the lines' and taking note of what is *not* said. This is most valuable if it can be backed up with other evidence. The relationship between latent and manifest content is circular; as one provides insights for the other, both may be analysed in one research project. Although latent content is based on subjective judgements, it can be quantified, although its richness will inevitably be reduced in the process.

Categorizing the data

Before analysing the data, researchers must decide how they should be categorized. Let us assume that you are interested in the ways in which disabled people are presented in the popular press, and have decided to analyse a random sample of magazine articles on disability and disabled people. The steps you should take are as follows:

1. Read the articles through and jot down all the ways in which disabled people are described. For example they may be described as pitiful, heroic, asexual, supernatural or 'normal'.
2. Decide whether any of the descriptions are so similar that they can be combined into one category.
3. Devise a simple chart (category frame) within which to record the various descriptions of disability. The categories must be exhaustive, which means that it should be possible to categorize every relevant item, and mutually exclusive, which means that no item can be recorded more than once. It is permissible to have an 'other' category, but this should be avoided if possible. It is very helpful, and can greatly improve reliability, if several people assist with the task of devising categories.

   A content analysis is no better than its categories. Reliability is greatest when categories are clearly stated and do not overlap. Too many categories reduce reliability because scorers cannot distinguish between them, but, on the other hand, highly reliable categories may lead to superficiality, reducing validity. Fine discriminations can be very difficult to code but may be extremely important; judges thought to be unreliable may be the most insightful. (For further discussion of reliability and validity, the reader is referred to Chapter 1.)

4. You will now need to decide how to analyse the data, if this was not decided in advance. Will you simply count the number of words which describe disabled people, or will you look for longer descriptions or themes? Will you take a positive description of disability at face value, or will you look for underlying meaning? Will you take pictures and photographs into account? Will you use specific measurements such as column inches?

5. You are now in a position to read the documents very carefully to analyse their content using the category frame. Write down any quotations which add substance to the data, and jot down any ideas and perceptions which may assist with your interpretation.

Reliability is improved if several researchers analyse the data. However, except in the most structured of analyses, for example word counts, researchers need a thorough understanding of the content to analyse it fully. (For further information on content analysis, the reader is referred to Krippendorff (1980).)

Documents used in documentary research

Any document, or visual or auditory material, is suitable for analysis by researchers. Below are some of the materials which may be used in documentary research.

Autobiographies and biographies

Autobiographies and biographies can provide an extremely rich source of data for researchers, including details of unusual personal experiences. They have the advantage of taking the individual's viewpoint into account and can provide an element of human interest which other research sources may lack. Autobiographies may also give the researcher ideas for the formulation of research questions and hypotheses. This is important as the meaning of a concept, such as disability, may be limited, leading to bias in the type of research undertaken and the type of knowledge produced.

When a large number of autobiographies on the same theme have been written, it is possible to make tentative generalizations which a single autobiography would not allow. A therapist interested in the coping strategies of disabled people, for example, may decide to read a large number of autobiographies on disability and carry out a content analysis. Although each autobiography will give an individual and highly subjective account of the experience of disability, the researcher may notice a few dominant coping strategies which are employed, or may be struck by the diversity of the coping strategies or the way they change over time.

The use of autobiographies and biographies in research does have limitations, however. For example, the authors are likely to omit various aspects of their story which might place them in a poor light or cause offence to others. Memories may be distorted, and it may be necessary to emphasize unusual or sensational aspects of the person's life in order for the book to sell, leading to bias in the information presented and, possibly, a blurring of fact and fiction. As Hammersley and Atkinson state:

> Authors will have interests in presenting themselves in a (usually) favourable light; they may also have axes to grind, scores to settle, or excuses and justifications to make. (1983:130)

The information in biographies is also likely to be distorted, in fact the author's motive in writing the biography may be to portray the person in the best possible light, perhaps in response to other biographies which have sought to discredit the individual concerned.

People who write autobiographies cannot be described as 'ordinary', most being either famous or having some unusual experiences to relate. It is simply not the sort of activity most of us engage in, even if we do feel we have something interesting to say. The task of writing an autobiography is also very time consuming and demands considerable literacy skills.

Diaries

There are various ways in which diaries may be used in research. If personal diaries are analysed the advantages and disadvantages are similar to those of the autobiography and biography. If diarists do not intend their material to be read, they may give a more honest account, although dishonesty and self-justification may still be present. Diaries have the advantage that they are usually written close in time to the events they record and thus suffer less than autobiographies and biographies from retrospective effects; nor are they distorted by the work of editors. Some diaries give very factual information, for example appointment diaries and log books.

Diaries can be useful in the study of private behaviour where observation is inappropriate or impractical. For example, a researcher may ask a group of people who are trying to lose weight to keep a diary recording the amount and content of the food they eat, and the type and amount of exercise they take. Alternatively, research participants, such as therapists, may be asked to record critical incidents or problems which they encounter at work. As with the questionnaire and interview, great care must be taken with the wording of questions, though sometimes participants may simply be asked to tick boxes in a grid every time a particular event occurs. Whatever the task, researchers must be sure that participants are able to carry it out and that they have the time and motivation to do so.

A disadvantage of this method is that researchers are obliged to rely on the motivation and accuracy of participants in keeping the diary. The fact that they have been asked to do so can also have a profound effect on their behaviour, thereby distorting the data. For example, if a researcher is interested in analysing a person's weight problem, this may, in itself, be sufficient to stimulate that person to lose weight. Used in this way, the diary cannot, therefore, be regarded as a truly unobtrusive research tool.

Researchers may also use diaries to collect their own primary data; this is common practice among those engaged in participant observation (*see* Chapter 12).

Newspapers and magazines

Newspapers and magazines provide a vast source of data on practically every topic, including health, illness and disability. However, they tend to concentrate on topical issues and there is frequent distortion as information is cut and rearranged; in addition, many national newspapers reflect a particular political angle. Such data would, however, be invaluable to therapists wishing to investigate lay concepts of health or illness. For example, they could analyse accounts of AIDS or cancer given in various popular newspapers and magazines, and perhaps compare these accounts with those in medical textbooks.

Professional journals

Although professional journals tend to be seen as objective and scientific, researchers should realize that many of the problems associated with newspapers and magazines apply equally to journals. Professional bodies are politically sensitive organizations, which can result in the rejection of papers which are critical of the profession, or which oppose an established view, regardless of their relevance, importance or standard. There may be a tendency to concentrate on a particular type of research, or only to publish statistically significant findings. All of this can lead to bias and will shape the knowledge produced in a particular direction.

Professional journals can, however, be of tremendous use to therapists undertaking documentary research. For example, by undertaking a content analysis of the last 5 years of a professional journal it may be possible to find significant trends, for instance in the attitudes of therapists towards psychiatric illness, or the use of a particular treatment approach. (For further detail of the distortions which can occur when research is published, readers are referred to French (1993).)

Essays

Stimson and Webb (1975) asked children to write essays concerning their feelings on going to the doctor. Similarly Neville and French (1991) asked physiotherapy students to write short essays on what they considered to be a 'good' or a 'poor' clinical experience. Therapists could use this method of research for any number of projects. For example they could ask disabled children to write of their feelings about therapy, or the difficulties they experience in mainstream school. The method does, however, favour articulate and literate people, and the content may be dramatized in an attempt to write a 'good' essay.

Official statistics

Official statistics are collected by the state and its agencies. Examples include the census, which is a questionnaire sent to every household every 10 years, and the registration of births, deaths and marriages. There is a great deal of statistical data available concerning health, illness and disability. Many official statistics are published annually and are readily available in libraries and book shops. Examples of these are *Social Trends* and *Regional Trends*. Unofficial statistics, perhaps those routinely gathered in therapy departments, can also be used in research.

It is important to comprehend the terminology when using official statistics. Many terms, for example 'illness' and 'disability', are difficult to define and may change over time and from place to place, making temporal and cross-cultural comparisons difficult. People are also sensitive to the social and political nuances of the time when responding to questionnaires. They may, for example, respond differently to questions concerning ethnicity now than they would have done 10 years ago, even though the question wording remains the same.

Official statistics provide a wealth of data but there is a great danger of viewing them as more reliable and objective than they really are. Statistics can be manipulated for political purposes, so it is important to ascertain who sponsored the study and what the research was for. If data produced are perceived to be politically damaging, they may be rejected or parts of them omitted or minimized. In addition, official statistics rarely reflect reality, for example the amount of crime reported is unlikely to tally with the amount of crime committed, and the amount of illness reported is a gross underestimation of the amount of illness which exists (French 1992b). Therapists using official statistics in their research should try to discover the sampling techniques used as well as the response rate obtained. If possible the recording instrument should also be scrutinized to determine its reliability and validity. As Irvine *et al.* state:

> All data, whether produced in the course of academic research or by state bureaucracies, are structured by the conceptual framework that is applied as well as by the technical instruments used in their production. It is the precise nature of these practical and theoretical commitments that needs investigating for each set of data. (1979:5)

(For further information on official statistics, the reader is referred to Irvine *et al.* (1979) and Slattery (1986).)

Advantages and disadvantages of documentary research

Documentary research has a number of distinct advantages when compared with some other research methods. It is relatively economical and largely unobtrusive, and enables researchers to analyse large amounts of high quality data which already exist. No other organization but government has the resources or the power to undertake such wide-ranging surveys as the census, and it is only surveys such as this which permit comparisons and trends over time and across cultures, or provide sufficient data for quantitative analysis of minority groups.

Documentary data also overcomes many ethical issues. For example, it may be possible to analyse people's reactions to a disaster without involving them in any way, and there is little need to go through ethics committees. Documentary research is not entirely divorced from ethical issues, however. As Homan points out:

> Data may be collected for an initial purpose which subjects regard as worthy, translated into statistical form and so stored, and then used for another purpose by a secondary analyst. (1991:90)

The disadvantages of documentary research are that it can be lonely, time-consuming and tedious to undertake, and is restricted to topics which have been spoken and written about. In addition documents may be distorted or may fail to reflect reality. (For further information on secondary analysis, the reader is referred to Hakim (1982) and Stewart (1985).)

Conclusion

Documentary research is not, perhaps, the first method that would spring to the minds of therapists eager to undertake research. It can, however, be very valuable, either as the sole research method or as one of many in a multi-method approach. It provides therapists with a vast array of ready-made, and often high quality, data, and provided a healthy scepticism is maintained, can be invaluable in answering various research questions. It provides an efficient and cost-effective way for therapists to engage in research.

This chapter is based upon French (1987a).

Chapter

14

Research Approaches

In this chapter the following five research approaches, where a range of research methods may be used, will be discussed:

1. The case study.
2. Longitudinal and cross-sectional research.
3. Action research.
4. Participatory research.
5. Triangulation.

The case study

Feuerstein describe the case study as 'a detailed description and anaysis of a single event, situation, person, group, institution or programme within its own context' (1986:48). A case study can involve a unit as small as an individual or as large as an entire community. It provides an opportunity to carry out an in-depth study of a unique event.

The case study was by far the most popular mode of clinical investigation during the first half of the twentieth century, but it fell into disrepute on the grounds of being unscientific. However, the case study is uniquely suited to the production of certain types of knowledge, and in particular to the development of theory. This realization, together with a growing number of critiques of 'scientific' and 'objective' research (see Albury and Schwartz 1982, Broad and Wade 1982, Boyle et al. 1984), has rendered the case study acceptable once more.

Case studies enable researchers to investigate indivduals or particular situations intensively over time, to produce data which would be missed or remain hidden in large scale studies. It is a flexible approach which enables researchers to take into account new information as it arises. Any topic can be chosen and any method or combination of methods can be used, including interviews, observation and the use of documentary evidence. Both quantitative and qualitative methods are appropriate; for example the researcher may carry out a series of highly structured observations of an individual, but later interview the same person in a relatively open-ended manner. Bell states that the case study 'is much more than a story about or description of an event or state. As in all research, evidence is collected systematically, the relationship between variables is studied, and the study is methodically planned' (1987:6).

The case study can be carried out during or after an event; the latter is often referred to as a case history. An example of a case history is that by Taylor (1977) who investigated the psychological health of a small community following a severe tornado. Frequently a number of case studies are combined in order to associate common themes or differences in outcome. An example of a multiple case study is that by Foster (1987), who investigated the process of institutionalization and de-institutionalization of people with severe learning difficulties.

Advantages of the case study approach

The case study is an excellent approach if the researcher requires a detailed understanding of a specific person or event. The aim may be to help plan an effective treatment programme or to develop a theoretical concept; in the former the results may be put into practice immediately. Although the knowledge produced relates to a particular person or instance, it can be enormously helpful to other people. With regard to therapists, Bailey states, 'Most of us have at least one client whose progress and style of learning could benefit others . . .' (1991:63).

The data produced in case studies can cast doubt on 'taken-for-granted' knowledge or theoretical assumptions.

Ponsford and French (1989) carried out a case study of a man who had learned to drive, and who earned his living as a driver, despite severe athetoid cerebral palsy affecting all his limbs. The stimulus to undertake the study was provided when the man, Mr T, drove a friend of his to a centre where driving instruction is given to disabled people. The staff of the centre, seeing Mr T and believing him to be a client, immediately felt pessimistic about his ability to drive.

The case study included a detailed physical examination of Mr T, tests of his physical and cognitive driving skills, observation, and an in-depth interview. Mr T's driving was found to be satisfactory in every respect, which threw doubt on the general assumption that people with severe physical impairments such as his cannot drive. Research methods which concentrate on groups of people miss unusual instances such as this. As Bell states, a successful case study provides a three-dimensional picture that will 'illustrate relationships, micropolitical issues and patterns of influences in a particular context' (1987:7).

This is one of the few research approaches available for investigating unique or unusual events, for example rare syndromes and medical conditions such as congenital indifference to pain, or unusual social situations. A famous case study is that described by Koluchova (1976), concerning twin boys who were kept isolated and almost totally neglected from the age of 18 months to 7 years. The subsequent rapid improvement in their abilities threw doubt on assumptions concerning the prognosis of seriously deprived and neglected children. It is not, however, a requirement that the topic of case studies be unusual or sensational; indeed a criticism of case study research is that it has tended to concentrate on sensational issues to the exclusion of the less dramatic.

The case study can provide preliminary data before the researcher embarks on a full-scale study, perhaps to accumulate knowledge before devising research tools such as the questionnaire. Case studies can also be a useful means of generating hypotheses and research questions. Conversely, the case study can be used after a large scale project is completed in an attempt to explain unusual or unexpected findings.

The opportunity to use many methods (a multi-method approach) is greater in the case study than in most other research approaches. The use of multiple sources of evidence strengthens the validity of the data and is strongly advocated by Yin (1984). Foster (1987) used documentary methods, interviews and observation in her multiple case research mentioned above. (The multi-method approach will be discussed later in this chapter.)

The case study approach may help to make the research process more democratic. In some ways it may be easier for 'non-researchers' or novice researchers to take part in case studies than in large scale research projects because they do not need to secure large amounts of funding and may be able to undertake the research as part of their everyday work. This is not to imply that case study research is particularly easy; Yin (1984) points out that it is difficult to make use of assistants in case study research because the studies cannot be regularized but rather depend on the ability to link theoretical issues to the data being collected in order to take advantage of unexpected opportunities and to interpret the information. In addition researchers must be adaptable and flexible with a sound grasp of the theoretical issues in question. They should also have knowledge of a wide variety of research methods. Yin states:

> No matter how the experience is gained, every case study investigator should be well versed in a variety of data collection techniques so that a case study can use multiple sources of evidence. Without such multiple sources, an invaluable advantage of the case study strategy will have been lost. (1984:92)

The results of case studies tend to be more comprehensive, intelligible and interesting to most people than more traditional research reports, which are frequently full of statistical tables, complicated graphs and jargon. Thus the case study approach assists in the dissemination of knowledge, helping to make it accessible to a wider audience. However, a shortcoming of case study research is that insufficient effort tends to be given to the formation of a comprehensive database which can be retrieved and scrutinized by interested persons. Such a database could include the researcher's notes, interview transcripts, observation schedules and important documents.

Limitations of the case study approach

It is often said that case studies are suitable for exploring or describing a situation but not for explaining it; there are certainly many uncontrolled variables which render causal explanations difficult to make. Herson and Barlow (1976), for example, believe that case studies do not allow us to make cause and effect conclusions. Yin, however, disagrees. He states that information from case studies can be used to 'explain the causal links in real life interventions that are too complex for the survey or experimental strategies' (1984:25).

Another frequently mentioned limitation of case studies is that the resulting data are specific to the particular case and therefore cannot be generalized to others. However, Cohen and Manion (1985) are of the opinion that case study data are, in practice, frequently used to establish generalizations in a wider context, and Bryman (1988) points out that quantitative research is, itself, frequently based on non-random samples. Generalization becomes possible if case studies are replicated and the validity of the data is strengthened by using a multi-method approach. More than one investigator can also be used in case study research to reduce the possibility of bias.

With regard to case histories, memory is notoriously unreliable, and selective. However, this criticism can be levelled against many research methods and is certainly not specific to the case history.

Longitudinal and cross-sectional research

Longitudinal research

In longitudinal research, the researcher repeats observations over an extended period of time, ranging from a few weeks to many years. Such studies might include the investigation of an organization's growth, the changing cognitive skills of a group of individuals, or the progress of patients receiving therapy. A sample of patients with stroke who received speech and language therapy from a specific hospital at a given time, for example, could be tested over a period of several years to investigate their progress. Many research methods may be used when conducting longitudinal research, for example interviews, questionnaires and observation.

It is essential, if a longitudinal study is contemplated, to determine how often the testing should take place. In the case of the patients with stroke, it may make sense to test them every 3 months, but if a researcher were investigating the career development of a group of therapists, a longer period of time between testing would be necessary. Similarly, a different time-scale would need to be adopted for patients according to their illnesses and impairments, as well as the stage of recovery they had reached; progress following a hip replacement, for example, is likely to be more rapid than progress following severe burns.

With longitudinal studies, it is vital that changes within the sample are seen within the context of wider extraneous changes. For example, the absolute decline in the number of children attending special schools may mean nothing when the overall reduction in the total number of school children, because of the reduced birth rate, is taken into account. If wider changes are not considered it is very easy to mislead and to become confused.

Cross-sectional research (correlational research)

Cohen and Manion state, 'A cross-sectional study is one that produces a "snapshot" of a population at a particular point in time' (1986:70). Cross-sectional studies attempt to examine processes over time by investigating *different* groups of individuals at *one* particular point in time. Thus, rather than investigating students through a course of study from beginning to end, information is gathered about groups of students (at one point in time) at various stages of the course – the first year, the second year, the final year and so on. The National Census is an example of a cross-sectional study in which large groups of people of different ages can be compared.

The topic under investigation does not necessarily have to focus on people. A cross-sectional study could be undertaken on the environmental effects of a pollutant by investigating, at *one* point in time, various water and soil samples which had been subjected to the pollutant for *different* periods of time. The method or methods chosen with both longitudinal and cross-sectional research will depend on the particular research questions posed, as well as practical considerations such as the availability of time and money.

What type of study should be used?

An example of a longitudinal study in a health context is that by Kemp (1988), who investigated the career paths of graduate nurses. Haak (1988), on the other hand, adopted the cross-sectional approach to study depression in student nurses during their training by taking a sample of students from each academic year at one particular point in time. Haak found, among other things, that 'burn-out' was most common among senior students.

A researcher wishing to undertake developmental research therefore has the choice of conducting a longitudinal or a cross-sectional study. For example, if a therapist was interested in the progress of patients with a particular condition during their stay at a rehabilitation centre, he or she could either conduct a longitudinal study of a given group of patients or a cross-section of patients could be taken. In the former case the study would last for the duration of the rehabilitation period, and in the latter case the progress and problems of each group could be compared: those who had been undertaking rehabilitation for 1 month, those for 2 months and so on.

Denzin (1970) is of the opinion that longitudinal and cross-sectional studies should be used together in the same piece of research. Like all research methods and approaches they each have advantages and shortcomings, thus the use of both approaches increases the validity of the findings, or if the findings conflict, it helps to develop new hypotheses. A therapist interested in the progress of patients following above-knee amputation, for example, may take a sample of patients at different stages of their recovery (the cross-sectional approach) but also investigate a small number of individual patients over a longer period of time.

Strengths and weaknesses of longitudinal and cross-sectional research

Longitudinal studies allow the researcher to examine changes in particular situations and particular individuals over time. Longitudinal research may reveal that one change, a new stimulating environment, for example, appears to bring about other changes, an alteration in the behaviour and mood of patients in psychiatric hospitals perhaps. Thus individual growth curves and patterns of behaviour can be seen. The fact that tests, observations, interviews and so on are repeated during the course of the longitudinal study helps to verify the validity of earlier findings. It is not, however, possible to be certain that the relationship between events is a causal one, as many uncontrolled variables operate.

With cross-sectional studies it is more difficult to make causal inferences, as the same people are not followed through, and the study takes place at one particular point in time. Any number of alternative explanations are, therefore, available. Kangas (1971) demonstrated that cross-sectional testing of intelligence showed a decline with age. This can be explained, at least in part, by the different social and cultural experiences of people in different age groups. Older people, for example, may have had less opportunity for a good education, which is known to influence IQ scores. In contrast to this, longitudinal studies show no decline in intelligence, as measured by IQ tests, at least until the age of 50, and probably later.

Therapists studying the natural course of various diseases by means of cross-sectional studies may also run into this kind of difficulty. They may, for example, find that a certain disease is most likely to occur in men during their sixth decade, and conclude that this is a biological aetiological feature of the disease. However, their findings may relate far more to social and cultural factors in the lives of men in that particular age range. One of the weaknesses of cross-sectional research, therefore, is the extreme difficulty of adequately matching the various samples under investigation.

Longitudinal studies tend to suffer from 'subject mortality'; the loss of research participants as time goes by. This leaves researchers with fewer representative samples than they originally had, particularly as those who drop out may not be typical of the participants as a whole. Cross-sectional research will not suffer from this disadvantage as the participants are tested just once. If a longitudinal study suffers badly from subject mortality, it is possible to top up the numbers by adding participants drawn from a similar cross-section of the community, although this does make the interpretation of findings very difficult.

It is easier to find volunteers for a cross-sectional study than a longitudinal study as it takes up less of their time. It has been found that people who volunteer to act as research participants do not represent a cross-section of the community (Silverman 1977), so it is likely that an even more specific sample would volunteer to become involved over a long time span.

Longitudinal studies do not typically involve large numbers of people, whereas cross-sectional studies often do. The restricted sample size of the longitudinal study may make it impossible for researchers to generalize their findings, but this will only be a disadvantage if generalization was what the researchers had in mind. The smaller the sample size, the richer the data are likely to be as there is more opportunity to gather in-depth information and to use a multi-method approach.

Another problem with longitudinal studies is that repeated research procedures – experiments, interviews, questionnaires – may change the behaviour of the participants, which will, in turn, threaten the validity of the findings. They may, for example, become practised in various tests and think a great deal about issues which would not normally interest them.

Due to continuous changes in thought and practice, as well as the replacement of researchers as time goes by, it is unlikely that longitudinal studies carried out over a long period of time will be completed in the way that was originally formulated. New ideas and theories may even invalidate completed work.

Although an attempt may be made to keep the measurements and procedures standard, this may prove impossible because of ethical considerations and changes in attitudes and language. Many of the experiments that were previously conducted on research participants are no longer considered ethical, and changes of attitude prohibit the use of certain words and phrases. For example it is no longer permissible to classify people with learning difficulties according to labels such as 'idiot' and 'moron', which was standard practice at the beginning of the twentieth century. It is well known that even small changes of language and wording are sufficient to alter the responses of research participants (Peabody 1961).

Douglas (1976) has pointed out that longitudinal studies avoid the duplication of background information, which has to be collected only once, and if an important issue is inadvertently omitted during one testing phase, the gap can be filled, to some extent, later on. This is not possible in cross-sectional studies as they typically involve fairly large numbers of participants who are not followed up.

Douglas (1976) also notes the flexibility of longitudinal studies, inasmuch as participants can be tested at turning points in their lives as they arise, for example following marriage, bereavement, or a change of career. It is possible to treat the participants of longitudinal research in this individualistic way because their numbers are often relatively small.

Longitudinal research is time consuming and costly, whereas cross-sectional research is comparatively swift and inexpensive. Researchers are often under pressure to complete research, and carry out many projects, in order to secure promotion and future funding. This mitigates against longitudinal research.

Action research

Action research has been defined by Cohen and Manion as 'an on the spot procedure designed to deal with a concrete problem located in an immediate situation' (1986:208). They believe that action research should be used 'wherever specific knowledge is required for a specific purpose in a specific situation' (1986:216).

In action research the role of the researcher is not that of a detached outsider, but rather an interventionist who is actively involved in planning, implementing, monitoring and evaluating changes in policy. The main aim of action research is to change practice or solve a particular problem within a given, practical context: the problem is never studied in isolation from the social setting which gives it meaning. Despite its down-to-earth orientation, action research frequently gives rise to new insights which help to develop theory.

The value of action research to therapists

Action research can be undertaken by a single practitioner. For example, a therapist may wish to solve a particular problem in his or her work situation, so will act as both clinician and researcher. Alternatively, a group of therapists may work together on an action research project, or one or more therapists may collaborate with non-clinical researchers. Since action research aspires to improve practice as its primary aim, rather than developing theoretical knowledge, findings are implemented quickly and research methods are modified as the research progresses.

Such a flexible and adaptable approach enables clinicians to pursue research as part of their clinical role and to focus on problems of immediate concern to themselves and their patients or clients. There are many practical problems in undertaking large scale research and these are made worse by the rigidity of large institutions such as hospitals. French (1983, 1986b) found many reasons why practising physiotherapists were inhibited from undertaking research, for example expense, lack of time and knowledge, and a greater interest in clinical work.

Action research is adaptable and flexible and can bring about change despite these constraints, although this does not mean that it is easy or involves no expense, or that co-operation on the part of those in authority is easily gained. Indeed, implementing the findings of action research can prove very problematic politically: the findings may, for example, go against an established practice or norm, or there may be resource implications.

Action research has an advantage over more traditional approaches in that it has the potential to implement solutions to problems quickly. Whitehead (1985) points out, when talking of teachers, that they tend to decry educational theory because it does not relate to their practical skills or their immediate concerns. It is likely that feelings such as these are also experienced by therapists. Action research is more systematic than a purely impressionistic gathering of information but, at the same time, the importance of practical and personal experience is recognized. As Bell states:

> The essentially practical problem-solving nature of action research makes this approach attractive to practitioner-researchers who have identified a problem during the course of their work, see the merit of investigating it and, if possible, of improving practice. (1987:5)

It may also foster in therapists a more critical approach and, through focusing on real life, clinically-orientated problems, encourage involvement in research. Another advantage for therapists is that they will not have to choose between clinical work and research, as the research is totally concerned with problems arising in the clinical situation.

Action research, applied research and evaluation research

There is much confusion among the terms 'action research', 'applied research' and 'evaluation research'. The distinction between them is not clear-cut and the terms are frequently used interchangeably. Sommer and Sommer, for example, define applied research as that which 'seeks practical answers to immediate problems' (1980:5), a definition which could apply equally well to action research. Cohen and Manion (1986) suggest that although both applied research and action research are scientific, action research is less scientifically rigorous in application of methods. Whereas applied researchers tend to be concerned with large, representative samples and the control of independent variables, those engaged in action research are more concerned with specific small scale problems located within a particular context. Smith defines evaluation research as:

> the assessment of the effectiveness of social programmes already put in practice which were designed as tentative solutions to existing social problems. (1975:293)

This evaluative element is, however, often part of action research and both 'action research' and 'evaluation research' can be subsumed under 'applied research' (Judd et al. 1991).

Participatory research

Participatory research is an approach to evaluation which has been evolving in recent years, particularly in the developing countries. Chambers refers to it as 'a new paradigm', 'a coherent and mutually supportive pattern of concepts, values, methods and action amenable to wide application' (1986:1). Participatory research aims to involve, at every stage of the research process (choice of topics, methods, evaluation and dissemination), those towards whom research is normally directed, people who Chambers describes as 'the last', for example rural village dwellers in developing countries, patients and disabled people.

There is no place for 'subjects' or passive co-operation in this approach, instead everyone involved is an *active* participant. The expertise and talents of everyone are utilized to the full and training is given if necessary; the approach does not, however, reject expert knowledge or help from outside, rather it aims to make traditional research more effective and more meaningful.

Any research method can be used, but the emphasis is on those which are eclectic, inventive and flexible, giving room for new ideas to emerge and allowing for changes of plan and direction as the research proceeds. Methods are adapted to suit the particular situation and the people involved, rather than squeezing ideas into a fixed method. With traditional research, complex issues are sometimes simplified or avoided because the methods are too rigid to accommodate them.

With the participatory approach most of the research is done in natural settings, rather than in the office or laboratory, with emphasis on implementation and action as an ongoing process, rather than on scholarly activity. Because of its flexible, pragmatic nature, participatory research has often been frowned upon by academics.

One aim of participatory research is to provide educational opportunities to those who are so often at the receiving end of research directed by 'experts'. This, it is hoped, will have the effect of increasing their skills, self-reliance and self-confidence, leading to social action which they perceive to be relevant. People are generally more committed if they take part in activities rather than being passive recipients; the researchers will also have much to learn from this approach.

Participatory research is a democratic means of accelerating social change and reducing exploitation. The widespread effects that Chambers (1986) believes participatory research may have are summarized below:

1. It breaks down the mystique surrounding research.
2. It balances grass roots and macro-analysis.
3. It ensures that the problems researched are perceived as problems by the community to which the research is directed.
4. It makes use of personal experience. Local and 'lay' knowledge are taken seriously.
5. It helps to develop self-confidence, self-reliance and skills in people to whom the research is directed.
6. It spans the cultures of academia and practice, thereby addressing both academic and practical issues.
7. It encourages democratic interaction and transfer of power, thus reducing exploitation.
8. It challenges the way knowledge is produced.
9. It gives a sense of collective responsibility.
10. It enables people to view their situation in a wider context.
11. It avoids the fragmentation of knowledge, providing a holistic approach.

12. It enables people to analyse their situation and take action.

Participatory research aims not only to investigate important issues but to facilitate fundamental social change. People at the bottom of any hierarchy rarely have sufficient power to generate knowledge, indeed such power is usually held by those furthest from the situation. As Brechin (1993) states, 'Research tends to be owned and controlled by researchers, or by those who, in turn, own and control the researchers'.

The result of this is that the issues investigated may have litle relevance to those to whom they are directed, thereby hindering meaningful social change. Some of the problems Chambers (1986) considers are associated with more traditional research approaches are summarized below:

1. Relevant modes of analysis are neglected. Methods tend to be rigidly adhered to and may determine both problem and solution.
2. The problems investigated may be of interest only to the researchers and other 'outsiders', and may be inappropriate to 'real' situations.
3. Traditional research tends to undervalue the people to whom it is directed by not enlisting their active involvement.
4. Action tends to follow published work, which is often out of date. Any action which follows usually depends on the judgement of 'experts'.
5. Traditional research tends to be costly.
6. The research is influenced by forces which favour the strong and powerful.
7. Certain issues are neglected because they are not the priority of any profession, thus gaps are left in the knowledge.

A shift of emphasis of the magnitude required to align traditional and participatory research would require enormous attitudinal and behavioural change on the part of those engaged in research. This is not to imply, of course, that traditional research is without its advantages, and that participatory research has no problems.

Relevance of participatory research to therapists

Participatory research may seem somewhat removed from the everyday world of the practising therapist, but this need not be so. A central theme of this approach is that practically everyone is capable of contributing to the research effort. Therapists, therapy helpers and patients may be reluctant to become involved in research, believing that enormous expertise is required and that it is best left in the capable hands of the 'experts'. Although it is true that some knowledge of research methodology is helpful, therapists and patients are at the sharp end of clinical practice and the knowledge they have gained through years of experience should never be underestimated or thought to be inferior to that of experienced researchers.

Therapists are also in a position to involve people who are often *researched* but who are rarely *consulted*; research into disability provides a good example. The way in which disability has been researched has become a major issue for disabled people and their organizations in recent times. In 1991 a series of seminars on the subject of researching disability were organized by disabled academics (Disability Research Seminars 1991), culminating in a conference (Researching Disability: Setting the Agenda for Change) in 1992.

Disability has generally been defined in an individualistic, medicalized way as an internal condition of the individual, and most research on disability, including the large Office of Population Censuses and Surveys (OPCS) government surveys (OPCS 1988a,b) reflect this orientation. Many disabled people, on the other hand, view disability in terms of social, physical and attitudinal barriers which could be removed if only the political will to do so were present.

If an individualistic stance is taken by researchers, then the questions posed will be based on impairment and not on discriminatory practices and lack of access. Oliver has reworded some of the questions used in an OPCS survey to illustrate this point. For example, in place of the question 'What complaint causes your difficulty in holding, gripping and turning things?', he substitutes the question 'What defects in the design of everyday equipment, like jars, bottles and tins, causes your difficulty in holding, gripping and turning them?' and in place of the question 'Did you move here because of your health problems/disability?', he writes 'What inadequacies in your housing caused you to move here?' (1990:7). Abberley believes that 'It is a political decision, conscious or otherwise, to employ questions of the first type rather than the second' (1991:158). The way in which disability is defined is a serious issue, as findings may be translated into practice (French 1992a,c).

Zarb (1992) draws a distinction between 'participatory research' and 'emancipatory research', believing that research cannot be emancipatory unless it is empowering, and that empowerment cannot be *given* but rather must be *taken*. Writing of research into disability he states:

> Participatory research which involves disabled people in a meaningful way is perhaps a pre-requisite to emancipatory research in the sense that researchers can learn from disabled people and vice versa, and that it paves the way for researchers to make themselves 'available' to disabled people – but it is no more than that. Simply increasing participation and involvement will never by itself constitute emancipatory research unless and until it is disabled people themselves who are controlling the research and deciding who should be involved and how. (1992:128)

Triangulation

The use of a single method when researching a complex issue, especially if it concerns human behaviour, is bound to produce research findings that are both limited and biased. In an attempt to solve this problem, Denzin (1970) advocates the use of a multi-method approach when researching complex issues. He terms this approach 'data triangulation'. A multi-method approach can be defined as the use of two or more methods when researching a given topic. It is more likely to capture the depth and complexity of a situation than a single method. As Shipman states, 'when one method only has been used there is a one-dimensional snapshot of a very wide and deep social scene' (1985:147). If two methods yield similar results researchers will have greater confidence in the validity of their findings because they are less likely to have been affected by possible limitations of the research methods themselves (Babbie 1992). Brewer and Hunter state that 'The multi-method approach is a strategy for overcoming each method's weaknesses and limitations by deliberately combining different types of methods within the same investigation' (1989:11).

Another important advantage of data triangulation is that it tends to break down divisions between research perspectives, for example 'experimental' and 'naturalistic' research or 'quantitative' and 'qualitative' research. In this way triangulation may help to remove prejudices concerning the relative value of various research methods. The knowledge gleaned from the use of different methods may sometimes conflict, which may give rise to new hypotheses and the development of theory.

Types of triangulation

Denzin (1970) has extended the concept of triangulation beyond methodology. He believes that time, space, theory, investigators, and levels of analysis, can all be triangulated.

Time triangulation

Most research projects deal with a problem or set of problems at one particular point in time, ignoring the possible effects that the passing of time may have on the research findings. In order to avoid this limitation, Denzin (1970) advocates the use of both cross-sectional research and longitudinal research in the same study.

In cross-sectional research time can be accounted for by using participants from different age groups. If it were found, for example, that people over the age of 45 were considerably less efficient at a given task than those under 45, it might be concluded that the passage of time had produced a deterioration in their performance. An alternative strategy, also taking time into account, is the longitudinal method where the same sample of people are tested over a period of months or years to gather data concerning changes in various characteristics and attributes, for example attitudes, personality, work status, health status or leisure pursuits. It was noted above that cross-sectional and longitudinal research can give opposite findings on the same issue, so the two methods can provide a check on each other.

Space triangulation

Most research is carried out within the confines of a particular culture or subculture, and yet the results are frequently generalized to wider populations. Space triangulation attempts to overcome this problem by drawing participants from diverse sectors of society. If the research findings are similar, despite social differences among the participants, then researchers will feel more confident about generalizing their findings. If, on the other hand, the findings differ according to the culture of the participants, then generalizations will not be justified. The data may, however, give rise to new and interesting hypotheses. A common criticism of psychological research is that much of it is carried out on psychology students, and then generalized, although psychology students do not constitute a cross-section of society. Using samples of patients in research is also problematic as people who consult doctors and therapists may not be a cross-section of people with any given disease or impairment (French 1992b).

Combined levels of triangulation

This refers to the use of more than one level of analysis. In a study of communication, for example, some researchers may be investigating how people communicate in face-to-face encounters, while other researchers may be investigating how the workings of large organizations affect communication. The first researcher is undertaking a 'micro' analysis of communication, whereas the second researcher is undertaking an analysis at a 'macro' level. Smith (1975) suggests seven levels of analysis which do, nonetheless, overlap: individual, interactive, organizational, ecological, institutional, cultural and societal. The level of analysis is often dictated by the subject discipline concerned; psychology and medicine, for example, largely concern themselves with the study of individuals, whereas sociology and anthropology have a much broader focus.

Each of these levels of analysis inevitably give a partial interpretation. For example, if a study is limited to the individual, then data relating to the individual's social network will not be taken into consideration. Even if the individual and his or her social network is studied, it is likely that wider societal, political and economic factors will be missed. By analysing problems at several different levels a more balanced analysis is likely to result, as well as possibly extending the theory on which the research was based.

Theoretical triangulation

Most research concentrates on one theory while ignoring competing theories. This leads to departmentalization of various research findings although the areas under investigation may be the same or very similar. Denzin (1970) advocates theoretical triangulation, in which researchers take competing theoretical positions into account in their research. In this way competing theories can be tested and links made between them, with the result that new insights may be gained and new theories developed. Such research is likely to involve collaboration with researchers from different fields and with diverse interests which, as well as extending knowledge, may break down prejudices.

Investigator triangulation

The involvement of two or more researchers, particularly if the methods used are qualitative, is likely to lead to more valid and reliable data. Research is a social act, with researchers having their own perspectives and biases which are likely to influence the research findings, even if the greatest care is taken to prevent this from happening.

Researchers with different perspectives, or from different professions or backgrounds, could deliberately work together on a research project. If they reached agreement, when observing a particular event or using a particular research tool, the likelihood of the data being both reliable and valid would be considerably increased, and if they did not agree this could give rise to new insights and hypotheses. Keith (1992) points out, with regard to research on caring, that only one version of a set of events has been studied (that of the carers), which has served to alienate disabled and elderly people by disregarding their experiences and viewing them as 'the problem'.

It may also be advisable to involve the participants of the research with the analysis of the data, for example the interpretation made by the researchers can be presented to the participants for their comments and, if they feel it is inaccurate, it can be amended. They may, alternatively, be regarded as full and equal members of the research team.

Methodological triangulation

Denzin (1987) divides methodological triangulation into two types: within method triangulation and between method triangulation.

Within method triangulation

Within method triangulation refers to the replication of research, a practice which is often neglected. It was noted in Chapter 11 that a result which is highly statistically significant may be achieved, but unless the research is replicated there is always the chance that the result is either due to chance or to limitations of the research method. If similar results are obtained when the research is replicated, researchers can be more confident in the validity and reliability of their findings.

Between method triangulation

Between method triangulation was discussed at the beginning of this section. It is the procedure whereby two or more methods are employed to answer a particular research question. A multi-method approach should not be used as an end in itself, but rather the methods should be carefully selected to throw light on the specific problem being investigated (Brewer and Hunter 1989).

Rubin and Babbie (1989) point out that triangulation deals with different potential sources of error in the various methods used. If the findings are similar despite different methods, for example the experiment, the questionnaire and observation, researchers can begin to have confidence that their findings are valid. For example if a therapist wants to discover the level of satisfaction felt by patients attending an out-patient clinic, he or she may give a large group of patients a questionnaire, carry out in-depth interviews with a smaller group, and observe the behaviour of another group in the out-patient department. The therapist may find that the results from the three methods tally but, on the other hand, it may be found that dissatisfaction was only expressed during the in-depth interviews, or that behavioural indicators of dissatisfaction, which were observed by the therapist, were never expressed. An attempt should be made to reconcile incongruous findings in an attempt to develop new hypotheses. (For further information on methodological triangulation, the reader is referred to Brewer and Hunter (1989).)

Disadvantages of triangulation

Despite the many advantages of triangulation, it is not very easy to implement because of its expense in terms of both time and money. In social research, for example, the questionnaire is very often chosen as the sole technique, not because the researcher is unimaginative or lazy, but because it is a relatively quick and inexpensive research tool to devise and use. Researchers may wish to carry out interviews, experiments and case studies but may find it quite impossible to do so.

Triangulation is not without its theoretical problems either; it was noted in Chapter 1 that research methods are rooted in philosophical frameworks which may not easily be linked together. If methodological triangulation is used as well as incorporating several other types of triangulation into the research, for example, space, time and theoretical triangulation, then the findings can also become prohibitive to analyse.

Therapists often undertake research in difficult circumstances, frequently incorporating it into their working day, and if they reject the whole notion of triangulation this is understandable, but they should be urged to think again; not all methods are expensive or time-consuming and the richness of the data which results is likely to compensate for all the hard work.

Conclusion

The particular research approach adopted by therapists will depend on their research questions and the conditions under which they work. Case studies and action research are most likely to appeal to therapists who wish to keep their focus firmly on individual patients, who want to understand their patients as individuals, and who like to put their findings into practice without delay. Practitioners often complain that the findings of large scale research projects and highly 'objective' research methods fail to help them find solutions to problems they encounter, or to improve the situation of those they seek to assist. Research which focuses on specific clinical issues and which aims to implement change in a short space of time are therefore likely to appeal to many therapists. As therapists frequently work with the same patients over a considerable period of time, longitudinal research in the clincial setting can also be both feasible and rewarding.

Triangulation is suitable when a holistic view of a complex situation is sought. It has the potential to bring competing theories, different researchers and diverse research methods together, which may result in the breakdown of prejudices as well as extending knowledge. The research findings may also be brought to a wider audience, especially if a variety of researchers with different perspectives are involved. This larger, more diverse readership may also be beneficial in the search for new ideas, as people are likely to interpret the findings in different ways according to their own experience.

Participatory research is part of a wider social movement concerned with equality and control by those at the bottom of the social hierarchy. Knowledge is power, and all the time marginalized people are excluded from the processes involved in the production of knowledge their position is unlikely to improve. Ways must be found of encouraging and enabling people to carry out research into their own situation, and for research practice to be adapted to ensure their full participation. Therapists have an important role to play in this social movement for equality.

This chapter is based upon French (1987b,c, 1988c–e).

Part Three

Reporting and Disseminating Research Findings

15

Writing a Research Report

Research reports come in many shapes and forms. You may be writing your report as a course requirement, in which case a great deal of detail will need to be given concerning the methods and procedures you used. Alternatively the research report may be written for the agency who funded your project. Research reports are also written for professional journals, newspapers, and groups of interested people, including your managers and the research participants who took part in your study.

Research reports will obviously vary considerably according to the readership; there is often a specific format you are required to follow which will be provided by tutors, funding agencies and journal editors. In this chapter the kind of research report required when studying for degrees and higher degrees will be considered, although much of what is said will also apply to other research reports.

Traditional research report

Title

You may well find that the title you chose at the start of your research project no longer seems appropriate when you come to write it up. This is because research is a dynamic process which rarely runs entirely smoothly. Some of your original ideas may, for one reason or another, have proved impracticable, and you are likely to have gained new insights as the research progressed, leading to unexpected changes of plan. Whatever the title of your research may be, it should be accurate, informative and not too long. Its accuracy will help those who are searching the literature in your particular area to ascertain whether or not your research is relevant to them.

Abstract

The abstract is a précis of your study, and although it appears at the beginning of the report it is usually written last. The abstract summarizes your study in just a few hundred words, enabling others to judge, without reading the entire report, whether or not it is relevant to their needs. The abstract should state your reasons for doing the research, the methods you used, and your main results and conclusions. It is vital that the abstract is clear, precise and informative. It may be necessary for you to provide a few key words in order for your study to be indexed.

Introduction

The introduction should 'set the scene' of your study, giving enough background information to place it in context and to provide a theoretical frame of reference. The introduction should contain the work of other researchers whose ideas relate to your own, or which puts your study in context. It is desirable that the research you cite is recent, although it may be appropriate to cite older research findings as a way of locating your study in a historical context. Seminal works from the past may also be included.

At the end of the introduction, you need to state your own research questions or hypotheses, the purpose of your study, and its relevance to clinical practice. It may also be necessary to state clearly the definitions of terms and concepts you intend to use, as these may have been defined in a variety of ways by other researchers; the concepts of 'stress' and 'health', for example, need careful definition.

Methods and procedures

In this section of your report, you should describe the research methodology and procedures you used in great detail. You should aim for sufficient clarity and precision to allow another researcher to replicate your study, although replication may be neither possible nor sensible with some qualitative approaches. The information you give in this section will depend on the nature of your study, but may include the following:

1. Details of the research participants: their age, gender, diagnoses, etc.
2. The size of your sample.
3. How you selected your research participants and what inclusion and exclusion criteria you used.
4. The research methods you used.
5. The data collection instruments you used, for example questionnaires, interview schedules, pieces of apparatus, observation schedules, etc.
6. The precise instructions you gave to research participants or research assistants.
7. Your sampling method.
8. How you coped with ethical issues, for example how you gained informed consent, whether or not you went through an ethics committee, how you protected research participants from possible harm, etc.
9. How you intend to analyse the data.

Brief details of your pilot study should also be given in this section.

Hicks (1988) suggests that the methods section should be divided into the following subdivisions:

1. Design.
2. Participants.
3. Apparatus.
4. Materials – questionnaires, interview schedules, etc.
5. Procedure.

Whether or not you decide to divide the methods section up in this way will depend on your particular study. Your guiding principles should be the comprehensibility of your report to readers, and the requirements of your tutors, funding body, etc.

The methods section should be relatively short and concise. If you have a great deal of detailed information which you consider to be important and relevant, it should be placed in the appendices.

Results

The results section should contain the 'facts' of your study. It is usual to begin with the more general results and then move to the more specific findings. If you have a lot of data you may need to be selective in what you present, but you should none the less ensure that it provides a well-balanced picture. It is appropriate to give a brief explanation of statistical tests in this section, although detailed statistical information is best placed in an appendix.

In order to assist comprehension, you should reduce your raw data to descriptive statistics, tables, graphs, pie charts, etc., making sure that they are labelled accurately and that a key of the symbols you use is provided. The results should be presented in such a way as to make them easy for the reader to assimilate and pleasant to read. It is important, however, that everything included in this section is there for a purpose. As Mann states, 'Tables of results are compiled to make a point not to make padding' (1985:211). Charts and tables should be explained verbally unless their meaning is very obvious.

Although most traditional research texts insist that the results section of research reports should be purely factual and separate from the discussion section, with some qualitative methodologies it is more sensible to combine the two. If, for example, themes from open-ended interviews are used to illustrate theoretical points, then it makes no sense to separate the results from the discussion and would be very confusing to the reader to attempt to do so (French and Sim 1993).

Discussion

In the discussion section of your report your results are interpreted and debated. Your findings should be placed in a theoretical context by relating them to the research highlighted in the introduction. You should discuss such questions as 'Do the results support previous research or contradict it?' and 'Do the results suggest alternative explanations or theories?'

You should make clear the limitations of your study in this section, as well as pointing out any major problems you encountered. Your sample may, for example, have been insufficiently large to allow generalizations of your findings to be made; the return rate of your questionnaire study may have been low; and a key person may have withdrawn at the last minute. Do not be ashamed or try to cover up mistakes or things that went wrong. As Kane states, 'Science advances by explaining what went wrong as well as what went right' (1985:176). If you are writing the research project as part of your course work, mistakes and shortcomings are unlikely to affect your grade, provided you own up to them. Grady and Wallston believe that making mistakes in research 'is encouraged and valued as an important way to learn and develop creativity' (1988:15), and Langley goes as far as to state that:

> Your research could be a complete disaster but you could still end up with a top grade if you clearly describe all the problems you had and show that you have learned from them. (1987:3)

This having been said, it is important not to overdo the reporting of misfortune and disaster, or to portray yourself as a victim or someone with an axe to grind.

There is no need to be alarmed if you cannot make complete sense of your data when writing the discussion. As Kane states:

> If you tried your best and can find no sense or pattern to some (or even all) of your results, say so. It may be that there is no sense or pattern, and you have made a contribution to the world by discovering that. (1985:176)

At the end of the discussion section you should point out the inferences which can be drawn from your research, its theoretical and practical implications, and the ways in which it could develop.

Conclusion

The conclusion can be written as a separate section or as a paragraph or two at the end of the discussion. It is important that any conclusions you draw really do result from your study, rather than from the work of others or what you *hoped* your study would reveal. The conclusion should highlight the main points of your research and emphasize those issues and controversies which you hope the reader will remember.

References

All the references you used in your study must be written in full so that interested persons can locate them without difficulty. There are many referencing systems from which to choose, but which ever one you use it is important to be consistent. With the Harvard system the names of authors with the dates are written in the text, with all the references listed alphabetically at the end of the study. Alternatively with the Vancouver system each reference is given a small number in the text and the references are listed at the end in the order of these numbers. You may also like to list the books and articles you found helpful in conducting your research, but which do not appear in your text. This listing can be headed 'Bibliography' and placed after your list of references. (For full details of various systems of referencing, readers are referred to French and Sim (1993).)

Appendices

Detailed information which would interfere with the flow of your text, or which only the more meticulous readers would wish to consult, should be located in the appendices which are placed at the end of your report. Even here it is important to be selective. Items suitable for inclusion include questionnaires, interview and observation schedules, raw data, letters, details of apparatus, details of statistical tests, and lists of organizations. According to the size of your study you may like to divide your appendices into various subsections, for example 'Appendix A', 'Appendix B', etc.

Lists of contents

When you have written the main body of your research report, your final task is to write a list of contents of the various sections, giving the correct page numbers. A list of tables and a list of figures (graphs, diagrams and pictures) should also be included, ensuring that the titles you give tally with the ones in the text.

Acknowledgements

You may like to acknowledge those people who have helped you to carry out your project successfully; these may include your tutor, the librarian, the research participants, the funding organization, or a relative or friend. This rarely needs to be more than a paragraph in length and should be placed immediately after the title, or right at the end of the report. It is customary to make it clear that you, as the researcher, are responsible for any errors or shortcomings in the study.

Further advice on writing a research report

Report format

Many research methodology texts provide a format for writing reports similar to that presented above. It is important to realize, however, that this standard procedure is not always appropriate and should not be used slavishly or without careful thought. The format you choose will, to some extent, depend on the nature of your research and your readership, as Kane states:

The academic disciplines, professions and business have developed conventions for organizing presentation. But if your audience falls outside these areas, there is no reason why you should use these particular standardized forms if something else makes sense and is useful. (1985:177)

The traditional research texts also advocate the avoidance of 'I' and 'we' when writing research reports, preferring a more formal approach. This convention is, however, gradually retreating as more and more people find such formality stilted, dull and pompous. This is especially so in qualitative research where the researcher is more involved with the research participants.

The writing process

It is necessary to allow plenty of time to write your report; several drafts will probably be necessary and good presentation is of the utmost importance. It is very helpful to get feedback on early drafts from other people, and to read other reports dealing with similar issues. References, in particular, need careful checking to ensure they are correct. It is vitally important that all the references you use, your notes, your ideas, and all the important documents you read, are stored carefully and methodically as you undertake your research. It is very irritating to lose an important piece of information when you come to write it up.

If you are writing your research report as a course requirement, you are likely to be given a maximum word allowance; it is important to adhere to this or you may throw marks away unnecessarily. Shortening a piece of carefully prepared text can be painful, but more often than not it is improved by the process. Generally speaking, the more open ended the research, the more difficult it is to write it up.

Many people feel inhibited about writing because they think they must start at the beginning of the document and work their way through sequentially to the end; this, however, is rarely necessary. It can be helpful, as a means of initiating action, to start with the easiest area; with the research report this tends to be the methods section because it is logical and factual. The abstract, in which you need to sum up the whole study succinctly, is usually written last. There is no need to wait until the study is complete before starting to write it up; the results section, for example, can be written when the data have been analysed. The introduction is best left until the study is complete as it is difficult to introduce a topic adequately before knowing precisely what it will contain, and further reading may be necessary as the research progresses.

It is becoming increasingly important that researchers avoid using language in their research reports which stereotype people and perpetuate false and damaging images. Researchers should endeavour to avoid sexist, ageist, racist and disablist language, as well as language which oppresses other minority and disadvantaged groups within society (Spender 1985, Gordon and Rosenberg 1989, Miller and Swift 1989, French and Sim 1993).

Presentation

The way in which your research report is presented is very important. Ensure that it is typewritten, in double line spacing with a clear type-face. Margins should be wide enough to allow tutors to comment, or for the study to be bound. Attention should also be paid to spelling, punctuation, the clarity of graphs and diagrams, and the accuracy of references. (For further advice on all aspects of writing, readers are referred to French and Sim (1993).)

Conclusion

Many people feel daunted by the prospect of writing up their research, but unless it is written up, and disseminated adequately, few people will know of its existence, and so will not be in a position to put the findings to use. The writing and dissemination of research findings should be considered an integral part of the research process which deserves just as much time and care as any other component.

16

Disseminating Research Findings

Successful dissemination is best achieved through competencies, charisma and stamina. (Osborn and Willcocks 1990:198)

Disseminating research findings is a neglected element of the research process; research participants, in particular, are often given little, if any, information. The dissemination of research findings is vitally important because unless they are made known they will be of little value. Partridge and Barnitt state:

Sometimes when you reach the end of your research and have written the report, you are heartily sick of the whole topic. Leave it for a month or so and then come back to consider papers and talks. (1986:91)

It is also important for our ideas to be critically analysed by others. As Brewer and Hunter state, 'The public clash of ideas is essential to the creative scientific process' (1989:179). There are three main ways of disseminating research findings:

1. Giving talks.
2. Writing for publication.
3. Posters.

Giving talks

Giving a talk about your research will come at the end of a much longer process of planning it; you should aim to make your talk interesting, stimulating and coherent. A verbal presentation of research normally includes a brief introduction, a statement of purpose, an account of methodology and procedure, a consideration of the major findings, and the researchers's own conclusions and recommendations.

If you decide to disseminate your research findings by means of a talk, careful consideration must be given both to its content and your presentation. The most important thing to remember is the audience: What is their particular interest in your research? What is the state of their knowledge on the topic? How does your research apply to their situation? Your talk will obviously be more difficult to prepare and present if people in the audience have different levels of knowledge, with some knowing nothing about the topic and others knowing more than you do. As Osborn and Willcocks state, 'Appreciation of audience needs is a prerequisite for adequate dissemination' (1990:195).

It is not usually satisfactory to read aloud from detailed notes when giving a talk. Reading verbatim from notes tends to sound dry and dull, and has the effect of distancing the speaker from the audience. It is best to talk in a clear, conversational style, keeping eye contact with the audience, and avoiding jargon and unnecessary detail. If you have had little or no experience of giving talks, you may, understandably, find the prospect of doing so without a detailed record rather alarming, but your performance will almost certainly benefit if you are sufficiently familiar with what you need to say to manage with the use of cards containing a few 'trigger' words or phrases. You can always keep your detailed notes close at hand for reassurance or emergency.

It is likely that your talk will be constrained within a strict time limit. This means that you will need to be very selective with regard to what you present, perhaps restricting yourself to one particular theme of your research. The most common mistake when giving a talk is to cram too much in; it is best to concentrate on the major themes rather than the detail. If you want to give more detailed information you can provide your audience with a handout or a reference list to follow up. It is best, when giving a talk, to speak a little slower than normal; verbalizing the talk to yourself, or recording it and playing it back, will help you judge the timing as well as building your confidence.

Whatever the length of your talk, it is vital that you hold the attention of your audience; the longer your presentation the more difficult this will be. One way of enhancing attention is to use a variety of audio-visual aids, for example slides, video and the overhead projector. All visual aids should be clear, simple, uncluttered and relevant, with an accurate match between their content and what is being said (Newble and Cannon 1989). It is also important that the needs of disabled members of the audience are taken into consideration, for example those with hearing or visual impairments (London Borough's Disability Resource Team 1991). Try to avoid giving the talk when people are likely to be inattentive, for example last thing on a Friday afternoon or at the end of a conference.

Another way of holding the attention of your audience, and increasing their enjoyment and satisfaction, is to encourage them to express their views and ask questions. Throwing the floor open to questions and possible criticism takes courage; a way of reducing the anxiety of this is to present your talk to some supportive but critical colleagues as a means of rehearsal. A further advantage of this is that it will provide you with feedback on your presentation and will help you to verify the timing of your talk.

To reduce unnecessary worry just before giving a talk, you should check all the equipment you intend to use and familiarize yourself with the room; if your talk is part of a conference it can be very reassuring to listen to an earlier speaker. Once you have started the talk, focusing your attention on the needs of the audience rather than on yourself can help to reduce anxiety. Be sensitive to their non-verbal communication, and make sure they can see the visual displays you present and hear you clearly. Do not be unduly concerned or embarrassed if you cannot answer every question you are asked, or if you agree with some of the criticisms made of your research. Never try to cover up errors or gaps in your knowledge; audiences usually respect honest, open speakers. As the presenter you are responsible for the overall mood of the group; a little humour can help you gain rapport with your audience, but only if it comes naturally to you. Some degree of anxiety is not a bad thing as it will stimulate you to give your best. (For further information on all aspects of teaching, the reader is referred to French *et al.* (in press).)

Publication

An important way of disseminating your research findings is to publish them in relevant journals and newspapers. The format for presenting your research will be similar to that of the research report (*see* Chapter 15), but the material will need to be far more condensed. Many journal editors will provide you with a 'contributor's guide' which will give details of the style and structure they require or prefer. Remember that journal editors work about 3 months in advance, so if you want your article to be published by a specific date it should be sent in good time.

Before presenting either your ideas or your work to a journal editor, it is essential that you carry out some thorough market research. You should write your article with a particular journal in mind and only present your ideas to an editor who is likely to be interested in them. Have a really good look at likely journals and magazines to see if your work is appropriate. Note the length and content of articles, the length of sentences and paragraphs, and the complexity of the language. It is vital to bear the readership in mind when deciding what to present and how to structure your article; a general readership would, for example, require a rather different approach to a readership of therapists.

When you have decided which journal to approach it is wise to talk to the editor about your ideas before proceeding to write, as a similar article may already have been accepted. Once your article is written, all you need to do is to send it to the editor with a covering letter. Attention should be paid to presentation; it should be typewritten or printed on A4 paper in double line spacing with generous margins.

In the case of professional journals, your article will go through a peer review system where it will be judged suitable or unsuitable for publication. More often than not you will be asked to make modifications and amendments; this period of negotiation, between the author and the reviewers, can be quite lengthy. With professional and academic journals, page proofs are supplied for authors to correct before the article is published; changes to the article will not be made without the author's permission.

With the more light-weight newspapers, the editor will normally decide whether or not to publish your work. If it is accepted you will be informed and it will appear in the newspaper a few weeks or months later. You will not normally receive proofs to correct and your article may be changed by the editorial staff without your permission. In this way research results are sometimes distorted.

Despite the possible distortion of your research findings when submitting them to the popular press, in many ways this is a more satisfactory way of disseminating research data, inasmuch as more people tend to read popular newspapers and magazines than prestigious, academic journals. Writing for the popular press is, however, rarely encouraged in academic and professional circles.

Posters

A popular way of displaying research findings at conferences is to design a poster, where the essential points of your research are displayed on a board attached to the wall. It enables interested people to look at the research in their own time, and to talk to researchers on a one-to-one basis. The size of the poster and details of presentation, for example the size of lettering, are usually stipulated by the conference organizers.

Space is obviously at a premium when designing a poster. What you display will depend on your particular research topic, but it will usually include the title of your project, the main reason for carrying it out, a brief description of the methods you used, your major results, and your conclusions and recommendations. It must look striking and interesting and be easy to read. The lettering should be more than 5 mm in height, and the text should be broken up with diagrams, photographs, graphs or pictures as appropriate. The use of colour can serve to enliven the poster. Desk top publishing software can be invaluable when constructing the poster, as can the help and advice of a graphic artist. Some poster displays also make use of other audio and visual exhibits which are relevant to the research, such as a short video, a tape recording, or an explanatory model. A handout or a list of references can also be provided.

Other ways of disseminating research findings

Feuerstein (1986) provides many other ways of disseminating research findings, especially in the context of participatory research where some people may be unable to read. These methods include the use of photographs, pictures and films. Cartoons can also be used to convey important information in a forceful and memorable way. Feuerstein explains how graphs can depict people and everyday objects, rather than symbols, to make them more meaningful.

Research findings can also be disseminated by means of audio-visual materials, training packs, booklets, radio and television, and meetings with individuals or pressure groups. Osborn and Willcocks believe that research can be appreciated by many different groups of people and state, 'An essential characteristic of good disseminatory practice is that boundaries are there to be broken . . .' (1990:198).

Dissemination of research findings should not necessarily be left until your project is complete, people can be kept informed by talks, newsletters, seminars and progress reports. The discussion which may arise from this can be invaluable to researchers in developing new ideas and insights.

Conclusion

Spender (1981) points out that, in a very fundamental way, ideas and research findings which are not in print do not exist. If you have completed a research project, no matter how small, or if you have some interesting ideas or experiences which may help or be of interest to others, try to distribute, publish or talk about them or your work and expertise will remain unknown by all but a few.

References

Abberley P. (1991) The significance of the OPCS Disability Survey. In Oliver M. (ed.) *Social Work, Disabled People and Disabling Environments*, Jessica Kingsley Publishers, London

Abberley P. (1992) Counting us out: a discussion of the OPCS disability surveys. *Disability, Handicap and Society*, **7(2)**, 139–155

Ackroyd, S. and Hughes J.A. (1981) *Data Collection in Context*, Longman, London

Albury D. and Schwartz J. (1982) *Partial Progress – the Politics of Research and Technology*, Pluto Press, London

Anastasi A. (1976) *Psychological Testing*, 4th edn, Macmillan, London

Anzul M. (1991) Reflecting. In Ely M. (ed.) *Doing Qualitative Research: Circles Within Circles*, Falmer Press, London

Atkinson D. (1993) Relating. In Shakespeare P., Atkinson D. and French S. (eds), *Reflections on Research in Practice* Open University Press, Buckingham

Babbie E. (1992) *The Practice of Social Research*, 6th edn, Wadsworth Publishing, Belmont, CA

Bailey D.M. (1991) *Research for the Health Professions*, F.A. Davis, Philadelphia

Bales R.F. (1950) *Interaction Process Analysis*, Addison-Wesley, Cambridge, MA

Bell J. (1987) *Doing Your Research Project*, Open University Press, Milton Keynes

Berger R.M. and Patchner M.A. (1988a) *Implementing the Research Plan: A Guide for the Helping Professions*, Sage, London

Berger R.M. and Patchner M.A. (1988b) *Planning for Research: A Guide for the Helping Professions*, Sage, London

Boyle C., Wheale P. and Sturgess B. (1984) *People, Science and Technology*, Wheatsheaf Books, Brighton

Brechin A. (1993) Sharing. In Shakespeare P., Atkinson D. and French S. (eds) *Reflections on Research in Practice*, Open University Press, Buckingham

Brewer J. and Hunter A. (1989) *Multi-method Research*, Sage, London

Broad W. and Wade N. (1982) *Betrayers of the Truth: Fraud and Deceit in Science*, Oxford University Press, Oxford

Brown R. (1988) *Group Processes*, Blackwell, Oxford

Bryman A. (1988) *Quantity and Quality in Social Research*, Unwin Hyman, London

Cadbury S. (1991) The experience of being a research student: what is it really like? In Allan G. and Skinner C. (eds) *Handbook for Research Students in the Social Sciences*, Falmer Press, London

Chambers R. (1986) *Normal professionalism, new paradigms and developments*, Institute of Development Studies Discussion Paper 227, University of Sussex, Brighton

Clegg R. (1982) *Simple Statistics*, Cambridge University Press, Cambridge

Cohen L. and Manion L. (1985) *Research Methods in Education*, 2nd edn, Croom Helm, London

Crawshaw J. and Chambers J. (1990) *A Concise A-Level Statistics*, 2nd edn, Stanley Thornes, Cheltenham

Delamont S. (1976) *Interaction in the Classroom*, Methuen, London

Delamont S. and Hamilton B. (1976) Classroom research: a critique and a new approach. In Stubbs M. and Delamont S. (eds) *Exploration in Classroom Observation*, Wiley, Chichester

Denzin N.K. (1970) *The Research Act in Sociology: A Theoretical Introduction to Research Methods*, Butterworth, London

Diener E. and Crandall R. (1978) *Ethics in Social and Behavioral Research*, University of Chicago Press, Chicago

Disability Research Seminars (1991) Policy Studies Institute, London

Douglas J.W.B. (1976) The use and abuse of national cohorts. In Shipman M.D. (ed.) *The Organization and Impact of Social Research*, Routledge and Kegan Paul, London

Doyal L. (1979) A matter of life and death: medicine, health, and statistics. In Irvine J., Miles I. and Evans J. (eds) *Demystifying Social Statistics*, Pluto Press, London

Faulder C. (1985) *Whose Body is it? The Troubling Issue of Informed Consent*, Virago Press, London

Fetterman D.M. (1989) *Ethnography Step by Step*, Sage, London

Feuerstein M. (1986) *Partners in Evaluation*, Macmillan, London

Flanders N.A. (1970) *Analyzing Teaching Behaviour*, Addison-Wesley, New York

Foster S.B. (1987) *The Politics of Caring*, Falmer Press, London

Fowler F.J. and Mangione T.W. (1988) *Standardized Survey Interviewing*, Sage, London

Francis A. (1988) *Advanced Level Statistics*, Stanley Thornes Cheltenham

French S. (1983) A study of physiotherapists as an occupational group – with special reference to their role in research. MSc Dissertation, London University

French S. (1986a) Handicapped people in the health and caring professions: attitudes, practices and experiences. MSc Dissertation, South Bank University, London

French S. (1986b) Researching the researchers. *Therapy Weekly*, **13(24)**, 6

French S. (1987a) In praise of the written word. *Therapy Weekly*, **14(3)**, 4

French S. (1987b) Action research: a flexible approach. *Therapy Weekly*, **14(3)**, 4

French S. (1987c) The multi-method approach. *Therapy Weekly*, **14(7)**, 4

French S. (1988a) How significant is statistical significance? *Physiotherapy*, **74(6)**, 266–268

French S. (1988b) The Delphi technique. *Therapy Weekly*, **15(16)**, 4

French S. (1988c) Long and short-term research methods. *Therapy Weekly*, **15(12)**, 4

French S. (1988d) Stating the case in point. *Therapy Weekly*, **15(14)**, 4

French S. (1988e) Dispelling the mystique surrounding research. *Therapy Weekly*, **15(18)**, 6

French S. (1992a) Defining disability – its implications for physiotherapy practice. In French S. (ed.) *Physiotherapy: A Psychosocial Approach*, Butterworth–Heinemann, Oxford

French S. (1992b) Why do people become patients? In French S. (ed.) *Physiotherapy: A Psychosocial Approach*, Butterworth–Heinemann, Oxford

French S. (1992c) Researching disability: a new approach. *Disability and Rehabilitation*, **14(4)**, 183–186

French S. (1993) Telling. In Shakespeare P., Atkinson D. and French S. (eds) *Reflections on Research in Practice*, Open University Press, Buckingham

French S. and Sim J. (1993) *Writing: A Guide for Therapists*, Butterworth–Heinemann, Oxford

French S., Neville S. and Laing J. (in press) *Teaching and Learning:*

A Guide for Therapists, Butterworth–Heinemann, Oxford

Fry E. (1986) *An Equal Chance for Disabled People*, Spastics Society, London

Galliher J.F. (1973) The protection of human subjects: a reexamination of the professional code of ethics. *American Sociologist*, **8**, 93–100

Glaser B.G. and Strauss A.L. (1967) *The Discovery of Grounded Theory*, Aldine, Chicago

Glastonbury B. and MacKean J. (1991) Survey methods. In Allan G. and Skinner S. (eds) *A Handbook for Students in the Social Sciences*, Falmer Press, London

Goffman E. (1968) *Asylums*, Penguin Books, Hammondsworth

Gordon P. and Rosenberg D. (1989) *Daily Racism: The Press and Black People in Britain*, Runnymede Trust, London

Grady D.E. and Wallston B.S. (1988) *Research in Health Care Settings*, Sage, London

Greer A. (1980) *A First Course in Statistics*, Stanley Thornes, Cheltenham

Groves R.M., Biemer P.M., Lyberg L.E., Massey J.T., Nicholls W.L. and Warsberg J. (1988) *Telephone Survey Methodology*, Wiley, New York

Haak M.R. (1988) Stress and impairment among nursing students. *Research in Nursing and Health*, **11**, 125–134

Hakim C. (1982) *Secondary Analysis in Social Research*, Allen and Unwin, London

Hammersley M. and Atkinson P. (1983) *Ethnography: Principles in Practice*, Tavistock Publications, London

Haralambos M. and Holborn M. (1990) *Sociology: Themes and Perspectives*, 3rd edn, Collins Educational, London

Harvey J. and Smith W.P. (1977) *Social Psychology: An Attributional Approach*, C.V. Mosby, St Louis

Henry G.T. (1990) *Practical Sampling*, Sage, London

Hersen M. and Barlow D.H. (1976) *Single Case Experimental Designs*, Pergamon Press, Oxford

Hicks C.M. (1988) *Practical Research Methods for Physiotherapists*, Churchill Livingstone, London

Hitch P.J. and Murgatroyd J.D. (1983) Professional communication and cancer care; a Delphi survey of hospital nurses. *Journal of Advanced Nursing*, **8**, 413–422

Homan R. (1991) *The Ethics of Social Research*, Longman, London

Honey J. (1989) *Does Accent Matter?* Faber and Faber, London

Huff D. (1973) *How to Lie with Statistics*, Penguin Books, Hammondsworth

Irvine J., Miles I. and Evans J. (eds) (1979) *Demystifying Social*

Statistics, Pluto Press, London

Jenkins R. (1987) Doing research into discrimination: problems of method, interpretation and ethics. In Wenger G.C. (ed.) *The Research Relationship*, Allen and Unwin, London

Jorgensen D.L. (1989) *Participant Observation*, Sage, London

Judd C., Smith E.R. and Kidder L.H. (1991) *Research Methods in Social Relations*, 6th edn, Holt, Rinehart and Winston, London

Junker (1960) *Field Work*, University of Chicago Press, Chicago. Cited in Hammersley M. and Atkinson P. (1983)

Kane E. (1985) *Doing Your Own Research*, Marion Boyars, London

Kangas J. (1971) Intelligence at middle age: a 38-year follow up. *Developmental Psychology*, **5**, 2

Keith L. (1992) Who cares wins? Women, caring and disability. *Disability, Handicap and Society*, **7(2)**, 167–175

Kemp J. (1988) A longitudinal study of nursing graduates. *Nursing Times*, **84(22)**, 53

Kerlinger F.N. (1973) *Foundations of Behavioural Research*, (2nd edn), Holt, Rinehart and Winston, London

Kimmel A.J. (1988) *Ethics and Values in Applied Social Research*, Sage, London

Kinsey A.C., Pomeroy W.B. and Martin C.E. (1948) *Sexual Behaviour in the Human Male*, W.B. Saunders, London

Kirk J. and Miller M.L. (1986) *Reliability and Validity in Qualitative Research*, Sage, London

Kirkham G.L. (1975) *Doc Cop*. Cited in Sommer R. and Sommer B.A. (1980)

Koluchova J. (1976) Severe deprivation in twins: a case study. In Clarke A.M. and Clarke A.D.B. (eds) *Early Experience: Myth and Evidence*, Open Books, London

Krippendorff K. (1980) *Content Analysis*, Sage, London

Laing R.D. (1983) *The Voice of Experience*, Penguin Books, Hammondsworth

Langley P. (1987) *Doing Social Research*, Causeway Books, Ormskirk

Lavrakas P.J. (1987) *Telephone Survey Methods*, Sage, London

Leach C. (1979) *Introduction to Statistics: a Nonparametric Approach for the Social Sciences*, Wiley, Chichester

Leget M. (1991) *An Author's Guide to Publishing*, 2nd edn, Robert Hale, London

Linstone H.A. (1975) Eight basic pitfalls: a checklist. In Linstone H.A. and Turoff M. (eds) *The Delphi Method: Techniques and Applications*, Addison-Wesley, Cambridge, MA

Linstone H.A. and Turoff M. (eds) (1975) *The Delphi Method:*

Techniques and Applications, Addison-Wesley, Cambridge, MA

London Borough's Disability Resource Team (1991) Access pack: an access guide to conferences and events for disabled people. Obtainable from Disability Resource Team, 127–133 Camden High Street, London NW1

McNeill P. (1990) *Research Methods*, 2nd edn, Blackwell, Oxford

Mann P.H. (1988) *Methods of Social Investigation*, Blackwell, Oxford

Marsh C. (1988) *Exploring Data*, Polity Press, Cambridge

Miller C. and Swift K. (1989) *The Hand-Book of Non-Sexist Writing*, 2nd edn, Women's Press, London

Morison M. (1986) *Methods in Sociology*, Longman, London

Morris J. (1992) Personal and political: a feminist perspective on researching physical disability. *Disability, Handicap and Society*, **7(2)**, 157–166

Nachmias C. and Nachmias D. (1981) *Research Methods in the Social Sciences*, Edward Arnold, London

Neville S. and French S. (1991) Clinical education: students' and clinical tutors' views. *Physiotherapy*, **77(5)**, 351–354

Newble D. and Cannon R. (1989) *A Handbook for Teachers in Universities and Colleges*, Kogan Page, London

Oakley A. and Oakley R. (1979) Sexism in official statistics. In Irvine J., Miles I. and Evans J. (eds) *Demystifying Social Statistics*, Pluto Press, London

Oliver M. (1990) *The Politics of Disablement*, Macmillan, London

Oliver M. (1992) Changing the social relations of research production. *Disability, Handicap and Society*, **7(2)**, 101–114

OPCS (1988a) *Disability Survey of Disability in Great Britain. Report 1. The Prevalence of Disability Among Adults*, HMSO, London

OPCS (1988b) *Disability Survey of Disability in Great Britain. Report 2. The Prevalence of Disability Among Children*, HMSO, London

Oppenheim A.N. (1966) *Questionnaire Design and Attitude Measurement*, Heinemann, London

Osborn A. and Willcocks D. (1990) Making research useful and usable. In Peace S.M. (ed.) *Research in Social Gerontology*, Sage, London

Ottenbacher K. (1986) *Evaluating Clinical Change*, Williams and Wilkins, London

Owen D. and Davis M. (1991) *Help With Your Project*, Edward Arnold, London

Owen F. and Jones R. (1990) *Statistics*, 3rd edn, Pitman, London

Parry A. (1991) Physiotherapy and methods of inquiry: conflict and reconciliation. *Physiotherapy*, **77**(7), 435–438

Partridge C. and Barnitt R. (1986) *Research Guidelines: a Handbook for Therapists*, Heinemann, London

Peabody D. (1961) Attitude content and agreement set in scales of authoritarianism, dogmatism, anti-semitism and economic conservation. *Journal of Abnormal and Social Psychology*, **63**, 1–11

Peace S.M. (1993) Negotiating. In Shakespeare P., Atkinson D. and French S. (eds) *Reflections on Research in Practice*, Open University Press, Buckingham

Peberdy A. (1993) Observing. In Shakespeare P., Atkinson D. and French S. (eds) *Reflections on Research in Practice*, Open University Press, Buckingham

Plummer K. (1983) *Documents of Life*, Allen and Unwin, London

Ponsford A. and French S. (1989) The man nobody thought could drive. *Therapy Weekly*, **15**(40), 9

Rees T. (1991) Ethical issues. In Allan G. and Skinner S. (eds) *Handbook for Research Students in the Social Sciences*, Falmer Press, London

Researching Disability: setting the agenda for change (1992). Conference. 1st June. Kensington and Chelsea Town Hall. London

Riddoch J. (1991) Evaluation of practice. *Physiotherapy*, **77**(7), 439–444

Rosenhan D.L. (1980) On being sane in insane places. In Mechanic D. (ed.) *Readings in Medical Sociology*, Free Press, New York

Rosenthal R. (1976) *Experimenter Effects in Behavioral Research*, Irvington Publishers, London

Rowntree D. (1981) *Statistics without Tears*, Penguin Books, Hammondsworth

Rubin A. and Babbie E. (1989) *Research Methods for Social Work*, Wadsworth Publishing, Belmont, CA

Sawyer H.G. (1961) The meaning of numbers. Speech before the American Association of Advertising Agencies. Cited in Smith H.W. (1975)

Scott J. (1990) *A Matter of Record*, Polity Press, Cambridge

Shakespeare P. and Atkinson D. (eds) (1993) Introduction. In Shakespeare P., Atkinson D. and French S. (eds) *Reflections on Research in Practice*, Open University Press, Buckingham

Shipman M. (1985) *The Limitations of Social Research*, Longman, London

Siddell M. (1993) Interpreting. In Shakespeare P., Atkinson D. and French S. (eds) *Reflections on Research in Practice*, Open University Press, Buckingham

Silverman I (1977) *The Human Subject in the Psychological Laboratory*, Pergamon Press, Oxford

Sim J. (1986) Informed consent: ethical implications for physiotherapy. *Physiotherapy*, **72(12)**, 584–586

Sim J. (1989) Methodology and morality in physiotherapy research. *Physiotherapy*, **75(4)**, 237–243

Slattery M. (1986) *Official Statistics*, Tavistock Publications, London

Smith H.W. (1975) *Strategies of Social Research*, Prentice Hall International, London

Sommer R. and Sommer B.A. (1980) *A Practical Guide to Behavioural Research*, Oxford University Press, Oxford

Spender D. (1981) The gatekeepers: a feminist critique of academic publishing. In Roberts H. (ed.) *Doing Feminist Research*, Routledge and Kegan Paul, London

Spender D. (1985) *Man Made Language*, 2nd edn, Pandora, London

Stewart D.W. (1985) *Secondary Research*, Sage, London

Stewart D.W. and Shamdasani P.N. (1990) *Focus Groups: Theory and Practice*, Sage, London

Stimson G.V. and Webb B. (1975) *Going to See the Doctor: The Consultative Process in General Practice*, Routledge and Kegan Paul, London

Stone S. (1991) Qualitative research methods for physiotherapists. *Physiotherapy*, **77(7)**, 449–452

Sullivan E. and Brye C. (1983) Nursing's future: use of the Delphi technique for curriculum planning. *Journal of Nursing Education*, **22(5)**, 187–189

Taylor V. (1977) Good news about disaster. *Psychology Today*, **October**, 93–94

Thorndike R.L. and Hogan E.P. (1977) *Measurement and Evaluation in Psychology and Education*, 4th edn, Wiley, London

Webb E.J., Campbell D.T., Schwartz R.D. and Sechrest L. (1966) *Unobtrusive Measures: Non-reactive Research in the Social Sciences*, Rand McNally, Chicago

Whitehead J. (1985) An analysis of an individual's educational development. In Shipman M. (ed.) *Educational Research: Principles, Policies and Practices*, Falmer Press, London

Williams F. (1993) Thinking. In Shakespeare P., Atkinson D. and French S. (eds) *Reflections on Research in Practice*, Open University Press, Buckingham

Yin R.K. (1984) *Case Study Research*, Sage, London

Zarb G. (1992) On the road to Damascus: first steps towards changing the relations of research production. *Disability, Handicap and Society*, **7(2)**, 125–138

Index